Francis G. Caro, PhD
Robert Morris, DSW
Jill R. Norton

Advancing Aging Policy as the 21st Century Begins

Advancing Aging Policy as the 21st Century Begins has been co-published simultaneously as *Journal of Aging & Social Policy,* Volume 11, Numbers 2/3 2000.

Pre-publication
REVIEWS,
COMMENTARIES,
EVALUATIONS . . .

"**A**N IDEAL TEXTBOOK for any graduate level course on the aging population. Stands out among existing books on social problems and policies of the aging society. SUCCINCT AND TO THE POINT. A must-read for students, researchers, policy advocates, and policymakers."

Namkee G. Choi, PhD
Professor, Portland State University,
Oregon

Advancing Aging Policy as the 21st Century Begins

Advancing Aging Policy as the 21st Century Begins has been co-published simultaneously as *Journal of Aging & Social Policy*, Volume 11, Numbers 2/3 2000.

The *Journal of Aging & Social Policy* Monographic "Separates"

Below is a list of "separates," which in serials librarianship means a special issue simultaneously published as a special journal issue or double-issue *and* as a "separate" hardbound monograph. (This is a format which we also call a "DocuSerial.")

"Separates" are published because specialized libraries or professionals may wish to purchase a specific thematic issue by itself in a format which can be separately cataloged and shelved, as opposed to purchasing the journal on an on-going basis. Faculty members may also more easily consider a "separate" for classroom adoption.

"Separates" are carefully classified separately with the major book jobbers so that the journal tie-in can be noted on new book order slips to avoid duplicate purchasing.

You may wish to visit Haworth's website at . . .

http://www.HaworthPress.com

. . . to search our online catalog for complete tables of contents of these separates and related publications.

You may also call 1-800-HAWORTH (outside US/Canada: 607-722-5857), or Fax: 1-800-895-0582 (outside US/Canada: 607-771-0012), or e-mail at:

getinfo@haworthpressinc.com

Advancing Aging Policy as the 21st Century Begins, edited by Francis G. Caro, PhD, Robert Morris, DSW, and Jill Norton (Vol. 11, No. 2/3, 2000). *"AN IDEAL TEXTBOOK for any graduate-level course on the aging population. Stands out among existing books on social problems and policies of the aging society. SUCCINCT AND TO THE POINT. A must-read for students, researchers, policy advocates, and policymakers."* (Namkee G. Choi, PhD, Professor, Portland State University, Oregon)

Public Policy and the Old Age Revolution in Japan, edited by Scott A. Bass, PhD, Robert Morris, DSW, and Masato Oka, MSc (Vol. 8, No. 2/3, 1996). *"Anyone seriously interested in the 21st Century and exploring means of adaptation to the revolution in longevity should read this book."* (Robert N. Butler, MD, Director, International Longevity Center; The Mount Sinai Medical Center, New York)

From Nursing Homes to Home Care, edited by Marie E. Cowart, DrPH, and Jill Quadagno, PhD (Vol. 7, No. 3/4, 1996). *"A compendium of research and policy information related to long-term care services, aging, and disability. Contributors address topics encompassing the risk of disability, access to and need for long-term care, and planning for a future long-term care policy."* (Family Caregiver Alliance)

International Perspectives on State and Family Support for the Elderly, edited by Scott A. Bass, PhD, and Robert Morris, DSW (Vol. 5, No. 1/2, 1993). *"The cross-cultural perspectives of the volume and the questions asked about what services are really needed and by whom they should be provided will be useful to the authors' intended audience in gerontological policymaking."* (Academic Library Book Review)

Advancing Aging Policy as the 21st Century Begins

Francis G. Caro, PhD
Robert Morris, DSW
Jill R. Norton
Editors

Advancing Aging Policy as the 21st Century Begins has been co-published simultaneously as *Journal of Aging & Social Policy*, Volume 11, Numbers 2/3 2000.

The Haworth Press, Inc.
New York •London •Oxford

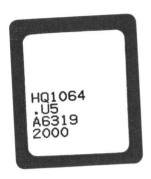

Advancing Aging Policy as the 21st Century Begins has been co-published simultaneously as *Journal of Aging & Social Policy*™, Volume 11, Numbers 2/3 2000.

The development, preparation, and publication of this work has been undertaken with great care. However, the publisher, employees, editors, and agents of The Haworth Press and all imprints of The Haworth Press, Inc., including The Haworth Medical Press® and Pharmaceutical Products Press®, are not responsible for any errors contained herein or for consequences that may ensue from use of materials or information contained in this work. Opinions expressed by the author(s) are not necessarily those of The Haworth Press, Inc.

The Haworth Press, Inc., 10 Alice Street, Binghamton, NY 13904-1580 USA

Cover design by Thomas J. Mayshock Jr.

Library of Congress Cataloging-in-Publication Data

Advancing aging policy as the 21st century begins / Francis G. Caro, Robert Morris, Jill R. Norton, editors.
    p. cm.
    Includes bibliographical references and index.
    ISBN 0-7890-1032-1 (alk. paper)–ISBN 0-7890-1033-X (alk. paper)
    1. Aged–Government policy–United States. 2. Aged–Government policy. I. Caro, Francis, G., 1936- II. Morris, Robert. III. Norton, Jill R.
HQ1064.U5 A6319 2000
362.6′0973–dc21
                                                            00-056707

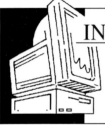

INDEXING & ABSTRACTING

Contributions to this publication are selectively indexed or abstracted in print, electronic, online, or CD-ROM version(s) of the reference tools and information services listed below. This list is current as of the copyright date of this publication. See the end of this section for additional notes.

- *Abstracts in Anthropology*
- *Abstracts in Social Gerontology: Current Literature on Aging*
- *Academic Abstracts/CD-ROM*
- *AgeInfo CD-ROM*
- *AgeLine Database*
- *Biology Digest*
- *Brown University Geriatric Research Application Digest "Abstracts Section"*
- *BUBL Information Service, an Internet-based Information Service for the UK higher education community <URL: http://bubl.ac.uk/>*
- *Cambridge Scientific Abstracts*
- *caredata CD: the social and community care database*
- *CINAHL (Cumulative Index to Nursing & Allied Health Literature)*
- *CNPIEC Reference Guide: Chinese National Directory of Foreign Periodicals*
- *Family Studies Database (online and CD/ROM)*
- *Family Violence & Sexual Assault Bulletin*
- *FINDEX, free Internet Directory of over 150,000 pubications from around the world www.publist.com*
- *GEO Abstracts (GEO Abstracts/GEOBASE) URL: http://elsevier.nl*
- *Health Management Information Service (HELMIS)*
- *HealthPromis*
- *Health Source: Indexing & Abstracting of 160 selected health related journals, updated monthly: EBSCO Publishing*
- *Health Source Plus: expanded version of "Health Source": EBSCO Publishing*
- *IBZ International Bibliography of Periodical Literature*
- *Index to Periodical Articles Related to Law*

(continued)

- *National Clearinghouse for Primary Care Information (NCPCI)*
- *New Literature on Old Age*
- *OCLC Public Affairs Information Service www.pais.org*
- *Referativnyi Zhurnal (Abstracts Journal of the All-Russian Institute of Scientific and Technical Information)*
- *Sage Public Administration Abstracts (SPAA)*
- *Social Services Abstracts www.csa.com*
- *Social Sciences Index (from Volume 1 & continuing)*
- *Social Work Abstracts*
- *Sociological Abstracts (SA) www.csa.com*

Special Bibliographic Notes related to special journal issues (separates) and indexing/abstracting:

- indexing/abstracting services in this list will also cover material in any "separate" that is co-published simultaneously with Haworth's special thematic journal issue or DocuSerial. Indexing/abstracting usually covers material at the article/chapter level.

- monographic co-editions are intended for either non-subscribers or libraries which intend to purchase a second copy for their circulating collections.

- monographic co-editions are reported to all jobbers/wholesalers/approval plans. The source journal is listed as the "series" to assist the prevention of duplicate purchasing in the same manner utilized for books-in-series.

- to facilitate user/access services all indexing/abstracting services are encouraged to utilize the co-indexing entry note indicated at the bottom of the first page of each article/chapter/contribution.

- this is intended to assist a library user of any reference tool (whether print, electronic, online, or CD-ROM) to locate the monographic version if the library has purchased this version but not a subscription to the source journal.

- individual articles/chapters in any Haworth publication are also available through the Haworth Document Delivery Service (HDDS).

Advancing Aging Policy as the 21st Century Begins

CONTENTS

ABOUT THE EDITORS

Francis G. Caro, PhD, is Professor of Gerontology and Director of the Gerontology Institute and Center at the University of Massachusetts Boston. He was formerly Director of Research for the Community Service Society of New York. He is co-author of *Personal Assistance: The Future of Home Care,* co-editor of *Achieving a Productive Aging Society,* and editor of the classic *Readings in Evaluation Research.* He is also a Fellow of the Gerontological Society of America.

Robert Morris, DSW, is Kirstein Professor Emeritus, Brandeis University, and Cardinal Medeiros Visiting Lecturer at the University of Massachusetts Boston, where he is Senior Fellow in the Gerontology Institute. He is co-editor of *Retirement Reconsidered* and *Welfare Reform: Is There a Safety Net?,* and co-author of *Personal Assistance: The Future of Home Care.* He is a past president of the Gerontological Society of America and has won several GSA awards.

Jill R. Norton, Editor/Publications Coordinator for the Gerontology Institute, University of Massachusetts Boston, was managing editor for this collection of essays. She also served in that role for the edited volumes *Achieving a Productive Aging Society* and *Older and Active: How Americans Over 55 Are Contributing to Society,* as well as for three previous Haworth Press, Inc. books.

INTRODUCTION

Advancing Aging Policy as the 21st Century Begins

Francis G. Caro, PhD

University of Massachusetts Boston

For reasons that go beyond the transition to a new decade, the year 2000 is a good time to give serious attention to the possibilities for aging policy development. In particular, in the United States, the economic and political climates have changed substantially in the past decade. Further, a new President will be inaugurated in January 2001. Symbolically, the beginning of a new decade and a new century also invite a review of the recent past and consideration of new possibilities. Through most of the 1990s, the climate for new public spending initiatives to benefit the elderly was unfavorable. The large federal deficits that had developed in the previous decade, a stubborn recession early in the 1990s, and major growth throughout the decade in expenditures for existing entitlement programs for the elderly lead to a narrow policy focus on cost containment. The political climate did not permit serious consideration of proposals for major new programs with significant cost implications. But late in the decade a combination of a dramatic improvement in the economy and containment of spending by the federal government resulted in a disappearance of the federal deficit as an immediate

[Haworth co-indexing entry note]: "Introduction." Caro, Francis G. Co-published simultaneously in *Journal of Aging & Social Policy* (The Haworth Press, Inc.) Vol. 11, No. 2/3, 2000, pp. 1-6; and: *Advancing Aging Policy as the 21st Century Begins* (ed: Francis G. Caro, Robert Morris, and Jill R. Norton) The Haworth Press, Inc., 2000, pp. 1-6. Single or multiple copies of this article are available for a fee from The Haworth Document Delivery Service [1-800-342-9678, 9:00 a.m. - 5:00 p.m. (EST). E-mail address: getinfo@ haworthpressinc.com].

1

public issue. Public officials are now debating about what to do with the surplus in federal tax receipts. Some new initiatives with modest public-spending implications that were unthinkable a few years ago can now receive consideration.

While the policy climate for aging issues has improved, policy entrepreneurs have good reason to proceed cautiously, however. Policymakers have been alerted to the fiscal implications of the impending retirement of the baby-boom generation. Proposals to put current surpluses into trust funds to postpone anticipated problems in financing Medicare and Social Security compete with proposals to use surpluses for new or improved benefit programs. Having learned about the cost containment problems posed by existing entitlement programs, policymakers are now very wary about new entitlement programs.

Policy advocates also have to contend with reduced public enthusiasm for public-sector initiatives, generally, and federal initiatives, more specifically. In an earlier period it was more plausible than now for policy entrepreneurs to propose federally financed benefit programs administered by a federal agency. Now, policy entrepreneurs have to emphasize less direct approaches. They are more likely to succeed at the federal level with approaches that encourage states, corporations, or private individuals to take certain specified actions. Approaches that provide tax credits are more likely to be embraced than those that require public expenditures. Particularly likely to gain favor in the current climate are mild public education initiatives that not only cost little but also have uncertain impact.

The range of aging policy issues receiving public attention needs to be broadened. In recent years, Medicare and Social Security have dominated the aging policy agenda. Income security and health care deserve center-stage attention because they rank at the top of the list of concerns of older people. Medicare and Social Security have commanded major attention also because of the challenges of sustaining the massive public financial commitments to them. Long-term care, housing, and transportation are conspicuous examples of other sectors of major importance to older people that deserve a more conspicuous place on the policy agenda. In an improved political climate, skillful entrepreneurs should be able to advance a wider range of aging policy issues.

Clearly, the opportunities and constraints in the policy environment in the United States cannot be generalized to the rest of the world. Nevertheless, other countries in the developed world are experiencing patterns similar to those in the United States. Some countries are preparing themselves for a rapid growth in the older population because they also have experienced a population surge after World War II. Some with strong social insurance programs that address income security and health care needs are now confronted with difficulties in containing costs as the number of older people covered continues to increase and health care becomes more sophisticated and costly. For these reasons, the international articles included in this collection reflect both similarities and differences in prospects for advancement in policies affecting older people.

We asked our invited authors to define for themselves what they considered advances in aging policy. In other words, we did not specify a framework of aging policy goals. Because we left open the question about what should be accomplished through policy, readers should be alert to the fact that the various authors have substantially different views regarding policy aims.

Authors were also asked to focus on what could be accomplished in the coming decade with consideration given to technical and political constraints. We suggested a relatively short-term horizon in the interest of encouraging attention to concrete options. We encouraged authors to emphasize feasible options rather than ambitious reform proposals that are not likely to receive serious consideration.

The collection begins with four essays concerned broadly with the potential for advancing aging policy. Scott Bass anticipates more favorable possibilities for aging policy because members of the baby-boom generation will choose in greater numbers to remain in the workforce. Through their workforce participation, older people will strengthen the economy. Businesses will increasingly appreciate the purchasing power of the more affluent older people who remain in the workforce. Bass anticipates a period particularly favorable for the older people with greater economic and social capital.

Robert Binstock makes the case for modest near-term political action to address the long-term problems faced by Social Security and Medicare. Binstock builds on the success of Social Security amendments of 1983 in strengthening the financial base of the program through modest adjustments that were not to be felt economically for many years to come. Binstock also calls for public education in terms that the general public can understand to strengthen the climate for public acceptance of political reforms.

By examining the United Nation's effort to develop a policy document as part of its celebration of the International Year of Older Persons, Charlotte Nusberg addresses the normative climate for attention to the needs of older people. She reports that thematic policy propositions which spoke to needs of people of all ages gained greater acceptance in the deliberations of United Nations representatives than did propositions explicitly focused on the needs of older people. The implication is that policy initiatives that will benefit older people may gain greater acceptance if they are embedded in initiatives that are beneficial to people of all ages.

Andrew Achenbaum examines the role that voluntary associations play in advancing the interests of older people. Achenbaum reminds us that voluntary associations have played major roles in civic life throughout the history of the United States. He traces the emergence of the "gray" lobby in the United States, assesses its strengths and weaknesses, and speculates about its future potential. Achenbaum, thus, demonstrates that the prospects for advancements in aging policy are likely to be influenced by the effectiveness with which the "gray" lobby develops and pursues its various agendas.

Four essays are concerned with employment of older people. Genevieve Reday-Mulvey makes the case for gradual or flexible retirement. Reviewing experiences throughout Europe, Reday-Mulvey argues that extended employment for older people on a reduced-time basis is beneficial for older people, for employers, and for pension systems.

Focusing on Germany, Winfried Schmähl makes the case for an extension of normal work life based on increased longevity. At the same time he calls for greater emphasis on retraining of older workers. Focusing on the United States, James Schulz argues for increased emphasis on training of older workers to protect them against the risks associated with economic change. Schulz reviews a number of promising strategies to strengthen the retainment of older workers.

Michael Barth addresses the implications of the growth of international markets for older workers. Barth argues that global markets are beneficial in spite of the challenges that they present to older workers. Barth advocates for employer investment in the upgrading of skills of older workers so that industries can remain competitive in the global marketplace.

Several authors have addressed diverse aspects of long-term care. John Nyman makes the case for expanded emphasis on continuing care retirement communities (CCRCs). Nyman is particularly sensitive to the assets tied up in homes owned by older people. He is critical of contemporary public policies that allow older people to retain ownership of their homes when they are permanent residents of nursing homes with Medicaid-financed care. Nyman prefers that older people draw upon their housing assets to finance their long-term care. Nyman argues that CCRCs are desirable from a public policy perspective because they encourage older people to sell their homes and use the proceeds to buy into a CCRC. In this way, older people draw on their own assets to help in the financing of their long-term care.

Masato Oka describes an unusual nursing home and community-based care program in Japan operated by a consumer cooperative. The organizational basis is a workers' collective whose members make both financial and service contributions. The approach is intriguing both because the worker association rather than the family or the government is the sponsor and the effort is based on a combination of financial and service contributions. The piece invites questions about the potential for replication of this approach elsewhere.

Robert Kane describes a new basis for organizing care of patients with chronic health care problems. He proposes that care be organized around the monitoring of "clinical glidepaths." They would provide a basis for establishing expectations for patient health that encompass a number of chronic conditions and offer the potential to permit better allocation, over time, of professional resources.

Andy Van Kleunen and Mary Ann Wilner call attention to the need for better training, compensation, and employment opportunities for long-term care workers, under both institutional and home care. They warn that unless these needs are addressed effectively, serious worker shortages will undermine the delivery of formal long-term care services. Van Kleunen and Wilner call for the federal government to take a variety of actions, including requiring better training of workers, changes in the reimbursement systems for Medicare and Medicaid to assure improved compensation for workers, and provisions to ensure better (*okay?*) health insurance for workers.

Iris Freeman examines the roles that regulators and consumer advocates play in advancing the quality of care in nursing homes. Freeman shows these roles are complementary. She argues that nursing home quality can be enhanced through a greater public investment in both inspection of nursing homes and consumer advocacy and stricter enforcement of standards.

Two essays address end-of-life issues. Amy Hutchinson and Henry Glick analyze the status and future of physician-assisted suicide and right-to-die policy options. In spite of the rapid emergence of physician-assisted suicide on the policy agenda, Hutchinson and Glick argue that it is not likely to be legalized in the near future in the United States. They observe that expanded emphasis on palliative care and hospice care are currently more acceptable strategies for dealing with end-of-life problems than physician-assisted suicide. Yet these authors are skeptical about whether the palliative care and hospice strategies will be sufficient and speculate that physician-assisted suicide will resurface on the policy agenda.

Dixon Sutherland and Rebecca Morgan discuss the collective difficulties in the United States in determining when to withhold treatment at the end of life. They call for an improved definition of death, more realistic policies concerning situations when medical intervention is futile, better alternatives than the courts in the resolution of conflicts around end-of-life cases, greater involvement of families in end-of-life decision making, and greater involvement of religious institutions in the development of policy options and in offering end-of-life ministry.

A range of other topics are considered in this collection of essays. Leslie Morgan addresses economic disadvantage and poverty among older women. Recognizing that the economic difficulties experienced by older women have multiple causes, Morgan outlines remedies in three sectors: Social Security, private pensions, and employment opportunity.

Jeff Yates and William Gillespie point to the dilemma of aging prison populations. A rapid increase in the number of elderly prisoners invites attention to cost containment, health care, and justice considerations. Yates and Gillespie review several strategies for dealing with the problem, including the segregation of older prisoners and an early-release program or "medical parole" for selected older prisoners. In addition, the authors call for age-based sentencing reforms or a restoration of judicial discretion in sentencing older criminals to restrict the number of older people in prisons.

Jan Mutchler and Jacqueline Angel address the policy implications of a large and rapidly growing Latino population in the United States. To help meet the needs of Latino elders, Mutchler and Angel call for improvement in the major entitlement programs: Social Security, Medicare, and Medicaid. They also speak to the need for service systems that are culturally sensitive and offer assistance in overcoming language barriers. To reduce future problems, they recommend investment in education and income support programs for younger Latinos.

Robert Hudson and Judith Gonyea discuss the potential offered by the Family Medical Leave Act in the United States. In an era in which the federal government was largely cutting back on its domestic programs, the FMLA stood out as a new measure to assist families struggling with health and long-term care problems. FMLA epitomizes the kind of largely symbolic intervention that was politically feasible during the recent past because it assured only unpaid leave. Hudson and Gonyea discuss the possibility that, in the period to come, the Act may be expanded to include paid leave–a modification with substantial implications.

Roger Cobb and Joseph Coughlin make a plea for attention to transportation. Reminding us that in this society the act of driving an automobile has become synonymous with transportation, they point out that transportation alternatives for those who do not drive are inadequate. The situation will only become worse with the growth in the older population–particularly in remote suburbs and rural areas. Cobb and Coughlin call for aging advocates, government, and industry to initiate a national dialogue to determine the role of government at various levels as well as the role of the private sector in addressing the problem.

Together, the essays in this collection provide strong support for the premises that led to this venture. They illustrate the wide range of important issues affecting older people that deserve attention from policymakers. The authors agree that the political and economic climate make it feasible to bring modest new initiatives with spending implications into the policy agenda. Further, the authors offer a variety of useful recommendations for advancing policy. My hope is that this collection will stimulate others to come forward with their own proposals for aging policy. Also useful will be efforts to develop more specific policy proposals and to test them against concerns about technical feasibility, cost, and political acceptability. In short, the essays provide a promising starting point for a constructive aging policy agenda in the period immediately ahead.

OVERVIEW

Emergence of the Third Age:
Toward a Productive Aging Society

Scott A. Bass, PhD

*University of Maryland
Baltimore County*

KEYWORDS. Productive aging, aging baby boomers, future aging policy, local aspects of aging policy

A possible future scenario of the policy context for older people in the United States that may unfold in the next decade will be explored in this essay. The challenges facing policymakers as we head toward 2010 will also

Scott A. Bass is Dean of the Graduate School and Vice Provost for Research at the University of Maryland Baltimore County (UMBC) and Distinguished Professor of Sociology and Policy Sciences. He has published extensively in the area of aging and social policy, including a 1995 edited volume supported by the Commonwealth Fund, *Older and Active* (Yale University Press). Dr. Bass was Founding Director of the Gerontology Institute and Center at the University of Massachusetts Boston. He can be contacted care of the Graduate School, University of Maryland Baltimore County, 1000 Hilltop Circle, Baltimore, MD 21250 (E-mail: bass@umbc.edu).

[Haworth co-indexing entry note]: "Emergence of the Third Age: Toward a Productive Aging Society." Bass, Scott A. Co-published simultaneously in *Journal of Aging & Social Policy* (The Haworth Press, Inc.) Vol. 11, No. 2/3, 2000, pp. 7-17; and: *Advancing Aging Policy as the 21st Century Begins* (ed: Francis G. Caro, Robert Morris, and Jill R. Norton) The Haworth Press, Inc., 2000, pp. 7-17. Single or multiple copies of this article are available for a fee from The Haworth Document Delivery Service [1-800-342-9678, 9:00 a.m. - 5:00 p.m. (EST). E-mail address: getinfo@haworthpressinc.com].

　　　　7

be considered. Aging policy as we know it, I believe, will need to undergo a substantial transition as we prepare for the entrance of elder baby boomers into the realm of senior citizenship. The political, economic, and lifestyle changes we have witnessed since the emergence of the baby boom in 1946 have been considerable. Based on the continuation of these trends, we can expect that their influences will have a significant effect on the way we think of aging and the aging society in the future (Rostow, 1998; Roszak, 1998; Torres-Gil, 1992).

Coupled with the expectations of the baby-boom generation, much of our policy context and many of our options will be influenced by the strength of our national economy. The working and spending habits of baby boomers are likely to sustain national economic growth which, in turn, will have unprecedented implications for public policy and public programs. It is further argued here that a sustained pattern of diminution of federal government involvement will intensify new issues at the state and local levels.

EMERGENCE OF THE THIRD AGE

The concept of the Third Age, a time period in one's lifetime between the completion of the primary family and traditional career responsibilities and old age and frailty, is being both defined and extended (Weiss & Bass, in press). The elements which better define the Third Age are emerging as we enter the new century. Pioneers among today's elderly are extending the frontiers of human potential in terms of their physical and intellectual activity in later life. Adults well into their seventies, eighties, and beyond are climbing mountains, exploring space, running marathons, writing books, managing corporations, building homes, and farming the land (Moody, 1988). Previously, retirement was considered to be a time of withdrawal, to make room for a younger and better-prepared generation, and of subsequent physical decline (Haber & Gratton, 1994; Riley, Kahn, & Foner, 1994). While leaders among today's elderly are beginning to question that concept, evidence is mounting that tomorrow's elderly will surely follow a different path.

Nevertheless, the Third Age is not just an extension of middle age or the sustained active engagement of those who were once considered the old. It is far more a transition of the institutions, norms, and opportunities afforded to older people as well; and, it is this larger societal transition–to new kinds of businesses, organizations, and enterprises–that the next decade will begin to foster. Matilda White Riley and her associates have been quite prolific about the structural lag of our institutions in their response to changing social behaviors (Riley & Riley, 1994). During the next decade, we will embark on this structural transition.

ECONOMIC GROWTH

Few people would have speculated 10 years ago that the start of the new century would be a time when the federal and state governments would be faced with decisions regarding budget surpluses–a time in which inflation would be nearly nonexistent, unemployment low, and welfare roles cut in half. Could they have imagined even the glimmer of reducing the federal debt, let alone any capacity for eliminating it? With the sustained economic expansion of the 1990s, such fantasies may become realities. Surely, our unprecedented economic growth may slow or even reverse itself; nonetheless, it does raise new ways to consider some of the concerns and fears associated with the costs of goods and services for the aging of the baby-boom generation.

If we had known in the 1930s of the huge birth spike between 1946 and 1964 that would cost the nation millions of dollars in hospital and health care and require new school construction, thousands of new teachers, and huge infrastructure costs, we would have said it was impossible for the nation to absorb such costs. From the perspective of a Depression era analyst, it would have been seen as a drain on federal, state, and local treasuries that would cripple the nation. In some ways, our lens on the demographic imperative–looking forward to the period 2020 to 2040, and very large numbers of older people–may be as imprecise. For the most part, the nation and its economy have successfully absorbed the early baby-boom era, most of which was expansionist. The dire consequences prognosticated regarding a growing, aging society may be just as unrealistic as it would have been in 1932 to forecast the economic consequences of the fertility boom that occurred from 1946 to 1964.

Much of our forecasting and planning for the aging society is based on a series of economic assumptions. These economic assumptions are largely accepted without critical examination. But, what if these historic middle-series assumptions are too conservative and actual growth exceeds projections, as witnessed at the end of the 20th century? What might the consequences be for the coming aging society and what are the implications for public policy? The Hudson Institute, a conservative think tank, in its report *Workforce 2020: Work and Workers in the 21st Century* explores a very different scenario for the future of aging than that of mainstream policymakers (Judy & D'Amico, 1997). For example, the Bureau of Labor Statistics projects that between 1996 and 2005, the United States will experience a one-percent-per-year labor-force growth rate (between 1996 and 1999, growth has exceeded those projections). This growth rate is lower, but is based on the actual 1.1% growth in the labor force experienced in America from 1982 through 1993. Rather than accepting this middle-series projection, the Hudson Institute report asks us to consider the implications of a slightly higher growth rate–say, 1.3% between 1996 and 2020, rather than 1% (Judy & D'Amico, 1997).

The consequences of a 1.3% growth rate would result in a demand for 11.5 million additional workers. Such a demand for labor would allow older workers, if they chose, to remain in the workforce and it would provide increased opportunity for other heretofore-surplus labor groups. Accompanying a growth in job opportunities, workers would have more money to spend, fueling economic growth and tax revenues while reducing the demand for public spending, including that on Social Security. According to the report, "Even if productivity does not accelerate, those millions of additional experienced workers could produce approximately half a trillion dollars of additional goods and services (in 1997 dollars) beyond what the national economy would otherwise produce" (Judy & D'Amico, 1997, p. 101). But, as we have seen in the economic cycles of the 1980s and 1990s, it is possible to have continued growth for long stretches that includes job expansion and increased productivity. Such growth creates considerable added wealth that fosters increased consumer spending. Economists refer to this phenomenon as the "wealth effect," in which people feel richer, have greater confidence in the future, and spend more. Active consumer spending, which constitutes nearly two thirds of the GDP, stimulates economic growth.

In the projected cycle of economic growth, the nation would be faced with rising tax revenues, revenues of $1 trillion beyond Congressional and Executive branch expectations, over the next 15 years. This $1 trillion surplus is based on a projected GDP growth rate of 2.4%. Between 1996 and 1999, the growth rate has been 4%. The rate of reduction of the nation's $3.7 trillion debt could be faster than projected, and the surplus could be even larger. By eliminating the national debt, interest rates would fall, allowing companies to borrow at favorable rates, and fuel further growth. With little or no debt by 2015, the United States, if it wanted to, could borrow to cover the costs associated with the aging baby boomers and once again retire the debt when the much smaller cohort of elders follows the passage of the baby-boom generation.

The same kind of calculations can be extrapolated to Social Security (OASDI Trustees Report, 1999). Most discussions about the Social Security Trust Fund are based on the intermediate estimate of GDP growth at 1.2% rather than the current 4%. As a result of this conservative estimate, it is projected that the surplus will disappear in 2034 and, at around 2014, Social Security will be paying out more in benefits than it receives in payroll taxes, requiring it to withdraw monies from the Trust Fund to make up the difference. An even more conservative estimate of growth reveals a dwindling Trust Fund by 2024. Nevertheless, there is a third estimate available that is less frequently discussed which anticipates a growth rate of 2.1%. Should growth be sustained at this level, there would be sufficient funds in Social Security to meet all obligations through 2075 without any alterations.

No one really knows what will happen with the economy, and it is important to develop cautious figures in planning for the future. It *is* possible that the economy could maintain the growth evidenced over the past 75 years, however; if so, the nation could afford an elderly society whose behavior in retirement is like that of previous cohorts. But, this essay argues that the upcoming cohort of elders will *not* behave like previous cohorts; and, as a consequence of the market behavior of the baby boomers, policy issues facing the ascendancy of the Third Age will be different from those of today.

BABY BOOMER BEHAVIOR

In national surveys conducted by the American Association of Retired Persons, baby boomers indicated that over three quarters of their cohort anticipate retiring by age 65 (Startch, 1998). This would leave a somewhat larger percentage working longer in their career jobs than people of the same age today. While many baby boomers may plan on retiring from their primary career jobs, a 1998 AARP/Roper survey indicated that four out of five boomer retirees plan to work during retirement (Startch, 1998); that is, after retiring from their lifetime career jobs, they intend to become engaged in some form of paid labor. The expectation of work after retirement is quite different than the expectations of today's retirees–fewer than one out of five individuals over age 65 is employed (Schulz, 1992). Indeed, the ravages of time may present another story; nevertheless, tomorrow's retirees are indicating that their retirement will be different than that of the previous generation. Over one third of the baby boomers in the AARP/Roper survey indicated they wanted to work part-time after retirement, primarily for interest or enjoyment.

Adults of the baby-boom generation are for the most part healthier, better educated, and wealthier than any previous American generation. The Congressional Budget Office compared real incomes (adjusted for inflation) and household size between baby boomers and their parents' generation. Depending on the age of the baby boomers, the income advantage (aggregate income and assets) of the boomers over their parents' generation at the same age ranged between 75% and 82% (Manchester, 1994). Even among lower-income baby boomers, their relative income was greater than the poor of their parents' generation. Still, among baby boomers, income inequality–the distance between affluence and poverty–is quite profound and, according to U.S. Bureau of Census figures, incomes in 1995 among baby boomers are more disparate than among the same age group 20 years earlier (AARP, 1998; Frey, 1999).

With more money and better education for the vast majority of baby boomers, baby boomers have had a significant effect on styles, fashions, and trends throughout their adult experience. From the sheer standpoint of economics and the capacity to spend, baby boomers should continue this behavior well into their retirement years.

For example, advertising in popular magazines is targeted at improving, masking, or altering the appearance of an aging body. Ads for "contouring facial lifts," removal of "wrinkles and brown spots," and vitamins to add vigor are already routine, and we have not yet entered the period of transition for baby boomers to the Third Age when all of this will accelerate.

Cosmetic surgery, once an exclusive choice of celebrities, has expanded dramatically. People are reconstructing entire bodies including noses, waistlines, breasts, eyes, and skin. In 1984, 477,700 plastic surgeries took place in America. This grew to 825,000 operations a decade later and continues to grow each year, driven by the demands of aging baby boomers. Interestingly, 65% of cosmetic operations were performed on individuals whose family income was below $50,000 (Sharlet, 1999).

Boomers will spend to look good and feel good despite their years; sometimes the products they buy will be fairly priced and of high quality and, at other times, they will not be. New pharmaceuticals will be developed and marketed to retard the maladies associated with human aging. Some book titles already attracting attention include: *Live Now, Age Later: Proven Ways to Slow Down the Clock, Immortality: How Science Is Extending Your Life Span–and Changing the World*, and *Living to 100: Lessons in Living to Your Maximum Potential at Any Age*. Unfortunately, many individuals fear their own aging and the implications of inching toward mortality. Rather than embracing the natural aging process, some older people will search for a fountain of youth at any cost.

Baby boomers will have more available in combined assets, pensions, and Social Security with which to retire than any previous generation; some will also experience financial windfalls in the form of inheritances. With about three quarters of the current population age 65 and older now owning their homes and 83% of these homes being fully paid for, baby boomers are most likely in line to inherit those properties. In 1987, the median value of all owner-occupied elderly housing was $58,900 (U. S. Bureau of the Census, 1990); this value has risen over the past decade. It is estimated that between 1990 and 2030, baby boomers will inherit $9 trillion (AARP, 1998). This windfall will help baby boomers continue their spending, which in turn will help the economy to grow, and sustain continuation of their social needs from the federal and state largess.

PUBLIC POLICY IN THE THIRD AGE

As we shift to an aging society in which 20% of the population is 65 or older, many of today's pressing issues of health care and Social Security may recede from the headlines to be replaced by new and different issues that focus on other work-related, invested interests of the able elderly. As the AARP Public Policy Institute (1998) notes, "Productivity gains, more than demographic changes, are key to the future economic prospects for boomers" (p. 58). The policy of the Federal Reserve Board and the behavior of the economy are crucial to the successful future of the baby-boom generation. Low interest rates and modest growth create demands for older workers; low unemployment with low inflation (a difficult balance) stimulates consumption that fuels the economy; a growing economy generates tax revenues to help pay for expansion of human services. A cycle of economic productivity that includes older people as part of the expanding economy is one in which the entire society benefits and one that can support the health and services needs of its dependent population.

Many issues other than health care and economic security will be determined outside of Washington, DC in the future. While we frequently think of Congress when considering public policy, many salient policy issues are of a state or local nature. In addition, the current conservative Supreme Court is proactive in asserting the independence of state governments and the reduction of federal authority. Two examples occurred recently. First, the Court ruled that a person who has a physical disability that can be corrected by medicines or devices is not disabled and therefore is not protected by federal law from discrimination; and second, the Court voted 5 to 4 to restrict Congress' authority to allow individuals to sue a state in state court to enforce their rights under federal law. In a time of shrinking federal power and a highly partisan Congress, public policy will continue to be made in the 50 state capitals and in local jurisdictions.

Some of the issues that older baby boomers will confront on a local level include land use, tax structure, transportation, environmental matters, workforce training, career counseling, volunteer programs, and housing. As boomers consider downsizing their residences, issues may be raised about the continued residential spread into rural communities, forcing the expansion of regional services and costly infrastructure. Alternatively, if baby boomers stay where they now live or consider moving closer to the urban core, greater environmental sustainability will be achieved. Discussion at the local level on regional policy in an aging society is a topic that will move to the forefront.

Indeed, concern about the housing patterns of retiring baby boomers may be a serious local issue. In his paper "Beyond Social Security: The Local Aspects of Aging America," William H. Frey examines the implications of a large, economically mobile, older population of baby boomers who are able to select the most desirable living environments, leaving city and county governments with uneven distributions of economically well-off elders and pockets of poor, older baby boomers in need of extensive public services. The current division between poorer-urban and more affluent-suburban neighborhoods will be revised; as a consequence of aging-in-place, large numbers of older people, unable to afford relocation, may become a strain on surrounding suburban neighborhoods. According to Frey (1999), "Concentrations of 'demographically disadvantaged' boomer elderly will arise within suburban communities that will not be prepared to deal with [their] social services, health care, and transportation needs . . ." (p. 3). With a larger elderly society that is more affluent and potentially less concerned about the needs of the poor, it may be that much more difficult to garner public support for programs at a federal level designed to mitigate these economic inequalities.

In the future, in a society in which older people will have a wide array of options and many will have the economic means to make choices, questions will arise as to the competitiveness and viability of many of the traditional, local aging organizations, such as the senior center. Senior centers, begun under the Older Americans Act of 1965 (OAA), now reflect a nationwide network of community agencies (Gelfand, 1999). These organizations face new competitors in the marketplace for older people's time and energy, including fitness centers, community colleges, restaurants, bookstores, and dedicated programs such as Elderhostel or lifelong learning centers. Created in a very different era, the OAA needs some retooling to reflect the needs of the aging society and to keep current with the changing interests and demands of older boomers. Two areas in need of immediate attention are (1) defining the role OAA can play in assessing and planning for flexible employment options for older people, and (2) providing incentives for OAA programs to upgrade their facilities, enhance their programs, explore partnering with the private sector, and revitalize their mission. Without these changes, the senior center and other allied OAA activities run the risk of becoming mere shadows of what they once were.

OAA was designed to serve all older people, regardless of income. With the greater choices afforded affluent elders and the speed with which the private sector can respond to fads for market segments, nonprofit or universal government programs may have a hard time competing for market share. Cumbersome rules and regulations may make these programs an option of last resort. Political support for OAA programs may decline, leaving only a core of constituents of modest economic means with modest services. Well-connected elders may focus their political clout on their own needs, which will be much more marketplace- and investment-oriented and less focused toward traditional, social welfare programs.

CONCLUSION

The next decade will be a period of transition wherein our society will move from policy directed at aging individuals to policies aimed at cultivating an aging society. Central to our aging society will be the nurturing of the nation's economy. A growing economy spells good years ahead for older baby boomers. Rather than being seen as liabilities, older baby boomers will be deemed assets with an important role in sustaining economic growth (see Roszak, 1998). If policies are crafted that tap the potential of baby boomers in the workforce, then it is likely we will experience unprecedented economic expansion. That is not to say, however, that there will not be poor and dependent elders; for there will be.

The experiences of a lifetime of low earnings are compounded for the aged through poor health, inadequate nutrition, poor dental hygiene, and the incapacity to solve situational financial problems. For these unfortunate elders, private charities and government funded organizations are the best hope. Government programs become their lifeline and support. Unfortunately, funding from these programs is likely to be modest. With a potential reduction in federal anti-poverty efforts, very poor and vulnerable elderly will be dependent on the services available in their immediate communities. Some elders will go without as considerable political clout will reside with more affluent elders. As pioneers of the aging society, attention will be given to the needs of these more organized and influential elders. In all likelihood, the vulnerable elderly will be dispersed geographically throughout suburban and urban areas and, for those who have aged in place in areas without a history of services, the capacity of those communities to meet their needs will be strained.

Despite the evidence of growing inequality, public policy will be driven by the economic interests of baby boomers. Most likely, legislation will be introduced that provides financial advantages to baby boomers. Bills will be focused on reductions in estate taxes, capital gains taxes, and mechanisms for older people to retain equity earned in their homes. Also, tax incentives will be proposed to provide long-term care insurance and mechanisms to foster individual solutions to high-cost health or long-term care expenses. These schemes will more likely follow the tax assistance historically provided to families for child care, with direct subsidies for long-term care for the very poor.

In the next decade, we will see new kinds of organizations, industries, and services to respond to the needs and desires of aging baby boomers. These new enterprises will require some regulatory and governmental oversight to ensure that consumers will not be defrauded or exploited. Public policy will be needed to develop regulations that are responsive, but not overly constraining, to these new industries. In a time of growing states' rights and shrinking federal authority, local decision making will be important to older baby boomers. Larger numbers of older people will require more cooperation among local jurisdictions to ensure coordination of local services. Regional planners will need to examine policies and programs to encourage housing and transportation patterns that are affordable and workable for local communities.

Finally, the OAA and the organizations it fosters will need to be updated to be responsive to the interests and habits of baby boomers. Areas in need of expansion and revision include local career training and employment options for the able elderly. Also, incentives will be needed to upgrade senior center facilities and provide activities that are more consistent and competitive with those found in the private sector.

The next decade will only usher in the transitional elements; the actual changes in organizations, structures, and initiatives will take place as the baby boomers move closer to traditional retirement ages in the second decade of the 21st century. Most important will be a sustained growth of the economy. Through continued economic growth, the country's middle-class aging baby boomers will experience a time of unprecedented prosperity.

REFERENCES

AARP (1998). *Boomers approaching midlife: How secure a future?* Washington, DC: AARP Public Policy Institute.

Bass, S. A., Kutza, E. A., & Torres-Gil, F.M. (1990). *Diversity in aging: Challenges facing planners & policymakers in the 1990s.* Glenview, IL: Scott, Foresman and Company.

Frey, W. H. (1999). *Beyond social security: The local aspects of an aging America.* Washington, DC: The Brookings Institution.

Gelfand, D. E. (1999). *The aging network: Programs and services.* New York: Springer Publishing Company.

Haber, C., & Gratton, B. (1994). *Old age and the search for security.* Bloomington, IN: Indiana University Press.

Judy, R.W., & D'Amico, C. (1997). *Workforce 2020: Work and workers in the 21st century.* Indianapolis, IN: Hudson Institute.

Manchester, J. (1994). *Baby boomers in retirement: An early perspective.* Washington, DC: Congressional Budget Office.

Moody, R. (1988). *Abundance of life: Human development policies for an aging society.* New York: Columbia University Press.

OASDI Trustees Report (1999). *1999 OASDI trustees report.* Washington, DC: Social Security Administration.

Riley, M. W., Kahn, R. L., & Foner, A. (Eds.). (1994). *Age and structural lag.* New York: John Wiley & Sons, Inc.

Riley, M.W., & Riley, J. W., Jr. (1994). Structural lag: Past and future. In M. W. Riley, R. L. Kahn, & A. Foner (Eds.), *Age and structural lag* (pp. 15-36). New York: John Wiley & Sons, Inc.

Rostow, W. W. (1998). *The great population spike and after.* New York: Oxford University Press.

Roszak, T. (1998). *America the wise: The longevity revolution and the true wealth of nations.* Boston: Houghton Mifflin Company.

Schulz, J.H. (1992). *The economics of aging* (5th edition). New York: Auburn House.

Sharlet, J. (1999, July 2). Beholding beauty: Scholars nip and tuck at our quest for physical perfection. *The Chronicle of Higher Education*, A15-A16.

Startch, R. (1998). *Boomers look toward retirement.* Washington, DC: AARP.

Torres-Gil, F.M. (1992). *The new aging: Politics and change in America.* New York: Auburn House.

U.S. Bureau of the Census. (1990). *Home ownership trends in the 1980s.* Current Housing Reports Series H-121, No. 2. Washington, DC: U.S. Government Printing Office.

Weiss, R.S., & Bass, S.A. (Eds.). (In press). *Challenges of the third age: Meaning and purpose in later life.* New York: Oxford University Press.

The Politics of Near-Term Action to Deal with the Aging of the Baby Boom

Robert H. Binstock, PhD

Case Western Reserve University
Cleveland, Ohio

KEYWORDS. Baby boom, old-age policies, older people, politics of aging, policy processes, American politics

From the enactment of Social Security in 1935 through the mid-1970s, American society constructed an old-age welfare state through which, in recent years, we spend about two fifths of our annual federal budget on programs benefiting older people.[1] Today, because members of the large baby boom birth cohort will begin reaching the old-age category in the decades ahead, responsible demographic and program expenditure projec-

Robert H. Binstock is Professor of Aging, Health, and Society at the School of Medicine, Case Western Reserve University. A former president of the Gerontological Society of America, he has authored and edited some 200 publications, most of them dealing with old-age policies and politics. The latest of his 20 books, co-edited with Leighton E. Cluff, is *Home Care Advances: Essential Research and Policy Issues* (New York: Springer Publishing Co., in press). Portions of this article are adapted from "Can We Shape the Future Now? Political Perspectives on the Policy Challenges of Our Aging Society," prepared for the conference Policy Options for an Aging Population, October 21-23, 1999, Leesburg, Virginia, sponsored by the Council on the Economic Impact of Health System Change (located at Brandeis University).

Robert Binstock can be contacted care of the Department of Epidemiology and Biostatistics, School of Medicine, Case Western Reserve University, 2222 Circle Drive, Cleveland, OH 44106 (E-mail: rhb3@po.cwru.edu).

[Haworth co-indexing entry note]: "The Politics of Near-Term Action to Deal with the Aging of the Baby Boom." Binstock, Robert H. Co-published simultaneously in *Journal of Aging & Social Policy* (The Haworth Press, Inc.) Vol. 11, No. 2/3, 2000, pp. 19-29; and: *Advancing Aging Policy as the 21st Century Begins* (ed: Francis G. Caro, Robert Morris, and Jill R. Norton) The Haworth Press, Inc., 2000, pp. 19-29. Single or multiple copies of this article are available for a fee from The Haworth Document Delivery Service [1-800-342-9678, 9:00 a.m. - 5:00 p.m. (EST). E-mail address: getinfo@haworthpressinc.com].

tions indicate that policy reforms are needed to maintain existing levels of government benefits for them in their old age. Yet, there are and will be many older people who–unable to do much to help themselves–need even more assistance than current government programs provide if they are to have an adequate level of well-being.

Although the economic and political challenges of sustaining (and perhaps improving) the old-age welfare state for the old age of baby boomers appear substantial, a number of politicians, policy analysts, commissions, committees, and organizations have generated proposals for dealing with them, as well as for expanding government support for financing long-term care. Some of these proposals call for incremental changes in existing programs and others are quite radical (e.g., Etheredge, 1999; Feldstein, 1999a; Feldstein, 1999b; Fuchs, 1999; Williamson, 1997), reflecting the present political milieu which is dominated by the themes of fiscal responsibility, personal responsibility, and reliance on the market (see Binstock, 1998). Yet, it seems unlikely that these proposals or alternative policy options will be adopted in the near term.

What might happen if action is postponed until most baby boomers have reached the ranks of old age? Various commentators have generated apocalyptic scenarios of the consequences of delaying action. Some have argued, for example, that it will be essential to set limits on health care for older people (e.g., Callahan, 1987). Others have suggested that aged baby boomers, in their self-interested pursuit of governmental benefits, will pose a fundamental threat to our political system (e.g., Thurow, 1996). Even if such apocalyptic visions prove to be far off the mark, our society may find it very difficult to ensure adequate levels of income, medical care, long-term care, and other supports for many aged baby boomers.

POLITICAL FACTORS AGAINST ADDRESSING
THE AGING OF THE BABY BOOM

If the political context of compassionate ageism and government expansionism that nourished the old-age welfare state (see Binstock, 1983) still prevailed, near-term policy actions to provide for older persons of the future would not be as politically difficult as they are today. But even if it that context existed, there are some perennial and contemporary political forces that would make such policy changes difficult.

The Aging of the Baby Boom Is Not an Immediate Crisis

Sustaining the old-age welfare state for aged baby boomers is not an immediate crisis. Meantime, elections are always imminent as crises for most politicians. So, their present attention to old-age policies is in terms of symbolic gestures and incremental proposals that they believe are important for positioning themselves favorably with the electorate. For example, we currently have the meaningless "lock box" politics of Social Security, in which members of Congress are acting as if spending a very small amount of the surplus that the OASI Trust Fund invests in government bonds would have a significant effect on the economy or on the long-term viability of Social Security. Attention to Medicare is focused on the incremental (but politically appealing) step of providing coverage for prescription drugs. And President Clinton has announced a very minor long-term care initiative that provides a negligible amount of financial assistance to a small number of people, coupled with some meagerly funded information and counseling programs (see Binstock & Cluff, in press).

Who Gains and Who Loses if Action Is Postponed?

Except for the rare individual who aspires to be a statesman–either in contemporary or historical perspectives–today's politicians would lose little, if anything, by failing to deal with the policy challenges posed by aged baby boomers several decades hence. Most of them will be long gone from public life when the chickens come home to roost. In contrast, if they support policy changes that are relatively radical and rather immediate enough to deal adequately with the aging of the baby boom, they could very well incur substantial opposition and retribution from older voters and other vested interests that have a substantial stake in the status quo.

The list of parties with vested interests in the status quo of the old-age welfare state is substantial. In addition to older people themselves, it includes the insurance industry, health care providers, long-term care providers, the "retirement living" industry, "elderly law" attorneys, financial counselors, pension funds, organized labor, the aging services network, to name some–and even AARP, which operates businesses with an aggregate revenue of several hundred million dollars for its more than 40 million members (see Morris, 1996).

On the other hand, some powerful vested interests would be supportive of policy approaches that involve substantial privatization of the old-age welfare state. Among them, of course, would be the financial securities industry and various kinds of financial counselors, as well as publicly held corporations that could anticipate aggregate new investments of hundreds of billions of dollars.

What about the vested interest of today's older voters in the old-age welfare state? After all, a ubiquitous journalistic cliché for warning politicians is that "Social Security is the third rail of American politics–touch it and you're dead!"

Empirically, however, this cliché has not held up because there are many fundamental reasons why older people do not vote in a cohesive fashion (see Binstock, in press). When old-age policy issues are prominent in presidential election campaigns (the arena most salient to old-age policies), the votes of older persons distribute among the major-party candidates in roughly the same proportions as do those of younger age groups (Binstock, 1997a). Even in the rare instances when it has been possible to differentiate substantially between candidates with respect to their old-age policy stances, no impact on older voters has been discernible. A classic case in point was Ronald Reagan's re-election in 1984. During the election campaign, Democrats portrayed him (with good reason) as having been an "enemy" of Social Security during his first term. Yet, in the balloting, older persons gave him 63% of their votes (as compared with 54% in 1980), slightly higher than the overall average and the proportions in all other age groups (Binstock, 1992).

Nonetheless, politicians behave as if older voters are a powerful political force. And this has important implications for the political feasibility of policy options that would involve a rather immediate change in the distribution of current old-age benefits in order to deal with aged baby boomers. Although older voters have not behaved cohesively, and old-age advocacy groups have not demonstrated a capacity to swing a decisive bloc of older voters, the *perception* of being powerful is, in itself, a source of political influence (see Banfield, 1961). Incumbent members of Congress are hardly inclined to risk upsetting the existing distribution of votes that puts them and keeps them in office. Few politicians, of course, want to call the "electoral bluff" of the aged or any other latent mass constituency, if it is possible to do so. Hence, members of Congress and their staffs take heed when their offices are flooded with letters, faxes, phone calls, and e-mail messages expressing the (not necessarily representative) views of older persons. And they provide AARP and other old-age organizations with ready access to policy discussions, even though these organizations have had little influence in the politics of enacting and amending major old-age policies (such as Social Security and Medicare) and have not prevented significant policy reforms perceived to be adverse to the interests of an artificially homogenized constituency of "the elderly" (Binstock, 1994; Day, 1998).

Yet, politicians remain wary of old-age organizations and "share [the] widespread perception of a huge, monolithic, senior citizen army of voters" (Peterson & Somit, 1994, p. 178). So they continue to court the votes of older persons, eager to capitalize on (and wary of) the possibility that their voting behavior may become more cohesive, and listen to the views of old-age interest groups despite their recent decline in political legitimacy (see Binstock, 1997b; Day, 1998). In electoral campaigns, politicians strive to position themselves on old-age policy issues in a fashion that they think will appeal to the self-interests of older voters, and usually take care that their opponents do not gain an advantage in this arena. And incumbents, of course, are especially concerned about how their actions in the governing process can be portrayed during the next campaign.

As a consequence, policy options for meeting future challenges, but involving rather immediate and relatively radical changes in the benefits that today's older persons receive, have little chance of adoption. With the aging of the baby boomers still a distant and abstract crisis, members of Congress are unlikely to endorse the following: cuts in current old-age income benefits; a risky privatization of current trust fund reserves, or other privatizing approaches; a drastic reorganization in the financing and/or delivery of Medicare; or an earmarked tax on older people to finance long-term care.

WHAT MIGHT ENHANCE ACTION ON POLICIES FOR AGING BABY BOOMERS?

Many of the proposals for substantial reform of Social Security, Medicare, and long-term care that have been put forth in recent years have received serious attention on the public policy agenda. But because of the political factors sketched out above, as well as for other reasons, there is little indication that they are likely to be adopted. What might make near-term adoption of such policies more possible?

Advance Planning, Distant Startup, and Gradualism

Today's politicians might espouse and support a policy option which, though enacted now, calls for changes that would take place in the medium-term future–and perhaps be implemented gradually from that point on. Such a policy would be unlikely to offend older or younger voters, and many of the various business and professional interests that are vested in the policy status quo would have sufficient time to adapt.

The Social Security Reform Act of 1983 provides an excellent illustration of this approach. Among other things, it enacted a change in the "normal retirement age" for full Social Security benefits, from age 65 to age 67. Yet, the change was not scheduled to begin until 20 years later, in 2003, and is scheduled to take an additional 24 years to be fully implemented–2027. This policy change elicited little outrage, unrest, or opposition, either from voters or from vested interests (such as employers, whose successors would have to pay more months and years of payroll taxes for whatever employees they might have in the future). In contrast, the portion of the Medicare Catastrophic Coverage Act of 1998 that required older persons to begin paying immediately out of their own pockets for insurance for extended hospital stays, at a rather steep rate, was repealed almost immediately following vociferous outcries from a minority of older persons (see Himmelfarb, 1995).

The change in Social Security's normal retirement age is a felicitous political model. It combined advanced planning with a far distant and gradually implemented policy change to deal with the aging of the baby boomers. Consequently, it engendered little opposition from old-age advocacy groups or any other parties. Unfortunately, from a policymaking point of view, the years when the baby boomers will reach old age are not now far distant. Yet, there is still some time left for the use of advance planning and gradualism to moderate political opposition.

Whatever policy options one has in mind, they will probably involve measures for increasing dedicated revenue. Following the 1983 model, a sales tax, a value-added tax, and/or even an increase in the payroll tax could be scheduled to begin some 10 or so years from now at miniscule rates. Then, the tax (or taxes) could be scheduled to increase very gradually over a number of years. Similarly, on the expenditure reduction side, upward changes in the age of eligibility for benefits, for instance, could also be phased in very gradually after a startup some years hence.

An approach of this kind is not sufficient, in itself, to enable a policy option to receive serious attention and possibly be adopted. Although the establishment of new revenue sources, for example, would be unlikely to incur much of an outcry from voters for whom the proposed changes would seem distant and relatively negligible, conservative politicians would be unhappy with the principle of "raising taxes." Employers would certainly oppose, say, an increase in their share of a payroll tax (although there is no inherent reason why the increase could not be confined to the employee share). And business and consumer groups could be expected to register opposition (although the distance and gradualism of implementation for such policies would be moderating factors). So, even if policy options to deal with the aging of the baby boomers incorporated features of advance planning, distant start-up, and gradualism–more would be needed.

"Crisis" as a Context for Getting Attention

At various times in American history, relatively radical social legislation has been politically feasible because the economic and social contexts of the time generated a sufficient sense of public crisis to overcome our endemic fragmentation of power and the many vested interests in the status quo. Certainly, the New Deal (though hardly comprised of a single, integrated policy option) was the product of such a sense of crisis. One might also argue that the Great Society programs were the product of a sense of crisis, whether that sense had its roots in the national reaction to the assassination of President Kennedy or in President Johnson's capacity to generate a sense of crisis concerning the plight of the poor and the social unrest in our inner cities–or both.

Perhaps near-term attention to an integrated old-age policy approach would be feasible if the aging of the baby boomers were more successfully marketed as a crisis. Although many policy analysts and elite commentators keep writing and speaking about the aging of the baby boom as a looming crisis in American society (e.g., see Peterson, 1999), there is little sign, if any, that the general public or even the media have engaged in the issues generated by the aging of the baby boomers, let alone in a crisis-like perspective. And this is understandable in the nature of the case–a far distant period portrayed by a lot of boring demographic and program expenditure projections.

Anthony Downs (1972) has argued that there is an "issue attention cycle" in American politics, rooted both in the nature of certain domestic problems and in the way major communications media interact with the public. With respect to the aging of the baby boomers, we are in what he terms the "pre-problem" stage of the cycle when the problem exists, " but has not yet captured much public attention, even though some experts or interest groups may already be alarmed by it" (p. 39). What does it take to move from the "pre-problem" stage to a "critical problem" stage? Downs suggests that "A problem must be dramatic and exciting to maintain public interest because news is 'consumed' by much of the American public (and by publics everywhere) largely as a form of entertainment" (p. 42).

How could the aging of the baby boomers be made more dramatic and more successful in the competition for news coverage? I am far from being an expert in communications and marketing, but I will sketch out one approach at the risk of seeming unsophisticated in this realm of affairs.

The fundamental strategy would be to undertake a media campaign that portrays the aging of the baby boomers as *a crisis for baby boomers, their families, and society–rather than a Social Security crisis and a Medicare crisis.* The central focus would be on *people rather than programs.* The key would be to convey the costs of policy inaction in terms of what it would mean tomorrow for older people, the nature of family obligations and lifestyles, and the fabric of familiar social institutions that are integral to daily life.

Such a campaign–perhaps undertaken by a President or some other political figure who can readily command media attention, or by some very well-funded organizational entity–should be strategically targeted to the 76 million baby boomers, and be strong enough to compete with advertising campaigns that tell this audience how to avoid growing old. Its initial goal should be to convey to baby boomers (perhaps in a congratulatory fashion) that they will live for many, many years as older Americans. (If old-age-related marketing to baby boomers seems far-fetched, we should be mindful that AARP is already engaged in it. Witness the recent special issue of *Modern Maturity* that pictured Susan Sarandon on the cover and featured a survey of the sex habits of Americans aged 45 and older [Jacoby, 1999].) Perhaps a complementary aspect of this first "congratulatory" phase would be to effectively inform baby boomers about the benefits of the old-age welfare state.

The next element would be to develop and convey scenarios that depict what life will be like for aged baby boomers if nothing is done to reconfigure the old-age welfare state and thereby sustain government supports at a level that is reasonably comparable to what older Americans have experienced in the last three decades of the 20th century. What will the budgets of elderly couples and aged widows be like in terms of how much they have to spend on food, shelter, clothing, utilities, transportation, medical care, and long-term care? Will some older persons have to be financially supported by their children? Will American society witness the return of three- and perhaps four-generation households? For those who are less than wealthy, what limits might exist on their access to medical care and high-cost, high-tech medical interventions, particularly at advanced old ages? In our increasingly long-lived society, how many baby boomers will be caring for or paying for the care of their functionally disabled parents who are of advanced old age? What will happen to the life-long savings of baby boomers who become functionally disabled and have no families to provide essential supportive personal care? For those who do not have adequate savings to pay for long-term care, or deplete them, and have no caring family, what can they expect in the way of help from government and the private and voluntary sectors of our society? And those who *have* families as caregivers? What will life be like for their caregiving (and often employed) spouses, siblings, adult children, and children-in-law, and perhaps their grandchildren? When "soccer moms" are transformed into unpaid nursing assistants engaged in endless caring? And on and on.

The generation and promulgation of scenarios that answer these questions might be enough to help baby boomers and their families feel that a sufficient "crisis" looms in societal support for the basic needs of older people to warrant policy action in the near-term future. If an issue as abstract, unfamiliar, and seemingly distant in consequences as global warming can reach the policy agenda, then near-term policies to meet the challenges of population aging surely could if the not-too-distant consequences are conveyed in terms of daily lives rather than projected program deficits.

If the scenery for the play of daily life in our aging society can be effectively painted for the American public, what else is needed to mobilize popular support for dealing with an aging society? As implied above, the daily issues confronting older people are not now, and will not then be, hermetically sealed from the rest of society. Perhaps the way to gain wide-spread political support is to paint an integrated policy option for an aging society as a "family policy" (see Harrington, 1999). If it proves to be effective, in many ways that is what–in effect–it will be.

CONCLUSION

Our capacity to respond adequately to the challenges of an aging society through governmental action is not dependent on sustaining the particular programs that were established through some four decades in which we constructed an old-age welfare state. Ultimately, of course, the fundamental issues are whether we will have sufficient economic resources to transfer to baby boomers in their old age, and whether we will have the political will to do so.

Twenty or 25 years from now, when most baby boomers will have reached the ranks of old age, our economy may not be prosperous. If we postpone until then the challenge of dealing with the aging of the baby boomers, confronting it may be economically and politically overwhelming. We might have a substantial crisis. The circumstances of daily life for older people might well resemble what earlier cohorts of older persons experienced prior to the construction of the old-age welfare state. Perhaps some of the apocalyptic visions of intergenerational conflict–class warfare between the young and the old–might come to fruition.

Although the adoption of a forward-looking policy may seem politically difficult at the moment, my view is that it can be done in the near future. We need to take advantage of the fact that we still (but not for long) have time to employ the strategy of a distant or semi-distant startup for new measures, with gradual implementation. We need to convey a sense of crisis, in a futuristic dimension, by focusing on the crises that will be entailed for people, not programs. And we need political leadership that can frame the issues of the baby boomers's old age in terms that enable us to understand that all of us–not just those of us who will be old at the time–will be affected. In short, if we can be brought to understand that "the beneficiaries 'R' us," we may have the political will to take action.

NOTE

1. Author's calculations, based on data in Congressional Budget Office (1999); Health Care Financing Administration (1998); Social Security Administration (1999).

REFERENCES

Banfield, E.C. (1961). *Political influence: A new theory of urban politics.* New York: The Free Press.

Binstock, R.H. (1983). The aged as scapegoat. *The Gerontologist, 23,* 36-143.

Binstock, R.H. (1992). Older voters and the 1992 presidential election. *The Gerontologist, 32,* 601-606.

Binstock, R.H. (1994). Changing criteria in old-age programs: The introduction of economic status and need for services. *The Gerontologist, 34,* 726-730.

Binstock, R.H. (1997a). The 1996 election: Older voters and implications for policies on aging. *The Gerontologist, 37,* 15-19.

Binstock, R.H. (1997b). The old-age lobby in a new political era. In R.B. Hudson (Ed.), *The future of age-based public policy* (pp. 56-74). Baltimore, MD: Johns Hopkins University Press.

Binstock, R.H. (1998). Personal responsibility and privatization in public policies on aging. *Public Policy and Aging Report, 9*(2), 6-9.

Binstock, R.H., & Cluff, L.E. (in press). Issues and challenges in home care. In R.H. Binstock & L.E. Cluff (Eds.*), Home care advances: Essential research and policy issues.* New York: Springer Publishing Company.

Callahan, D. (1987). *Setting limits: Medical goals in an aging society.* New York: Simon and Schuster.

Congressional Budget Office (1999). *The economic and budget outlook: Fiscal years 2000-2009.* Washington, DC: U.S. Government Printing Office.

Day, C.L. (1998). Old-age interest groups in the 1990s: Coalitions, competition, and strategy. In J. Steckenrider & T. Parrott (Eds.*), New perspectives on old-age policies* (pp. 131-150). Albany, NY: State University of New York Press.

Downs, A. (1972, Summer). Up and down with ecology–the "issue-attention cycle." *The Public Interest, 28,* 38-50.

Etheredge, L. (1999). Three streams, one river: A coordinated approach to financing retirement. *Health Affairs, 18*(1), 80-91.

Feldstein, M. (1999a). Common ground on Social Security. *New York Times,* March 31, A29.

Feldstein, M. (1999b). *Prefunding Medicare.* Cambridge, MA: National Bureau of Economic Research, Working Paper 6917.

Fuchs, V.R. (1999). Health care for the elderly: Who will pay for it? *Health Affairs, 18*(1), 11-21.

Harrington, M. (1999). *Care and equality: Inventing a new family politics.* New York: Alfred A. Knopf.

Health Care Financing Administration (1998). Medicare and Medicaid statistical supplement, 1998. *Health Care Financing Review,* statistical supplement.

Himmelfarb, R. (1995). *Catastrophic politics: The rise and fall of the Medicare Catastrophic Coverage Act of 1988.* University Park, PA: Pennsylvania State University Press.

Jacoby, S. (1999). Great sex: What's age got to do with it? *Modern Maturity, 42w*(5), 40-45, 91.

Morris, C.R. (1996). *The AARP: America's most powerful lobby and the clash of generations.* New York: Times Books.

Peterson, P.G. (1999). *Gray dawn: How the coming age wave will transform America–and the world.* New York: Times Books.

Peterson, S.A., & Somit, A. (1994). *Political behavior of older Americans.* New York: Garland.

Social Security Administration (1999). Current operating statistics. *Social Security Bulletin, 62*(2), 108-148.

Thurow, L.C. (1996, May 19). The birth of a revolutionary class. *New York Times Magazine,* 46-47.

Williamson, J.B. (1997). A critique of the case for privatizing Social Security. *The Gerontologist, 37,* 561-571.

Towards a Society for All Ages

Charlotte Nusberg, AARP
Washington, DC

KEYWORDS. United Nations, age integration, public policy, international, International Year of Older Persons

"Towards a Society for All Ages" was the theme chosen by the United Nations (UN) to celebrate the International Year of Older Persons in 1999. The theme, though ill-defined, could be interpreted as moving us away from a narrow focus on problems of the elderly towards a more holistic perspective encompassing all generations, perhaps as a counterbalance to the many UN conferences of the last few decades that have focused on special groups or concerns. I believe the theme was chosen as much in the realization that a narrow focus on older persons would not appeal to policymakers and the public in many parts of the world, as from an awareness that a holistic approach might just make better social policy sense.

The selection of the theme was the culmination of almost two decades of notable lack of political will among member states of the UN to move ahead forcefully on implementing the recommendations of such seminal documents as the Vienna International Plan of Action on Aging, adopted in 1982. This neglect was fueled in part by other urgent priorities and the lack of significant

---

Charlotte Nusberg is Coordinator for International Information at AARP, and serves as the International View Editor for the *Journal of Aging & Social Policy*. She also served as Secretary-General of the International Federation on Ageing and as the editor of *Ageing International*. She can be contacted care of the AARP Research Information Center, 601 E Street, NW, Washington, DC 20049 (E-mail: cnusberg@aarp.org).

[Haworth co-indexing entry note]: "Towards a Society for All Ages." Nusberg, Charlotte. Co-published simultaneously in *Journal of Aging & Social Policy* (The Haworth Press, Inc.) Vol. 11, No. 2/3, 2000, pp. 31-39; and: *Advancing Aging Policy as the 21st Century Begins* (ed: Francis G. Caro, Robert Morris, and Jill R. Norton) The Haworth Press, Inc., 2000, pp. 31-39. Single or multiple copies of this article are available for a fee from The Haworth Document Delivery Service [1-800-342-9678, 9:00 a.m. - 5:00 p.m. (EST). E-mail address: getinfo@haworthpressinc.com].

31

material support on the part of the UN and other international organizations. It should come as no surprise that those UN agendas that are accompanied by financial and technical assistance stand a better chance of being implemented than do their not so well endowed counterparts.

I was approached by a leading member of a UN planning committee for the Year of Older Persons to try to develop a document that addressed the theme and might be adopted by the General Assembly to honor the Year. The good news is that such a document was developed in broad consultation with older persons and their representatives all over the world. The bad news is that UN delegates, in their wisdom, seem to have concluded that the world no longer needs more documents addressing social issues and seems unlikely to endorse any statement as part of the Year's activities. Rather, the emphasis is on urging the implementation of existing plans and strategies.

However, *Strategies for a Society for All Ages*[1] now exists as a global discussion document for the Year issued by the organization I work for–AARP, an American non-governmental organization representing older persons. I believe it does provide policy directions for decisionmakers in governmental and nongovernmental institutions to build a more equitable society that moves us towards a society for all ages–one in which the interests of the young, middle-aged, and old are protected and promoted. A number of countries, in fact, are for the first time developing national plans on aging this year and seeking guidance from others.

A society-wide perspective is presented, both in the belief that this is the soundest strategy for moving "Towards a Society for All Ages," and in the hope that such an approach will resonate more with the public and policymakers. The *Strategies* have, in fact, been used by groups in many countries as part of their discussions for the Year and, in several, as a catalyst for action.

WHAT ARE THE STRATEGIES?

The *Strategies* are a series of 42 recommendations addressed to the institutional players of society–that is, governments, employers, trade unions, educational institutions, nongovernmental organizations, and so forth in both developed and developing countries. They are designed to be suggestive rather than prescriptive, in the hope of stimulating dialogue about what steps need to be taken to reach a society for all ages. While all the *Strategies* may not be relevant to the heterogeneity of social and economic circumstances in which nations find themselves, our hope is that users will select and prioritize those strategies that do currently make sense, revisiting the remainder at some future time.

The *Strategies* are organized into three sections linked by the common theme of interdependence–the interdependence of life stages, the interconnectedness of generations, and the interdependence of individuals and society. Interdependence came to be the framework for the *Strategies* in order to: (1) give some meaning to the concept of a society for all ages; (2) develop a unique document suitable for 1999 and beyond that moved the dialogue about aging forward by taking a more holistic approach; and (3) highlight and reaffirm some of the excellent thinking already reflected in previous UN action plans by interweaving this work with the conceptual framework for the Year.

The organizing principle of interdependence came about through a rereading of some of the seminal documents already enacted by the General Assembly over the last few decades–notably the Vienna International Plan of Action on Aging and the UN Principles for Older Persons enacted in 1982 and 1991, respectively. While these were ostensibly developed with older persons in mind, what was striking was how many of the recommendations were relevant to all age groups. This reinforced the fact that not only did older persons share many of the same needs and concerns that people of all ages face, but that by limiting policies to older persons as we sometimes do with our categorical programming, we ignore similar needs in the larger population. Where this occurs, the seeds are sown for a possible resentment among generations.

Thus, an important criterion for the selection of the *Strategies* was that they played an important role in improving the lives of all persons, regardless of age. But because, after all, the *Strategies* were being prepared for the International Year of Older Persons, an additional criterion imposed was that the *Strategies* be particularly important for achieving a quality old age.

The hope was that the *Strategies* would provide a valuable opportunity to reflect on our interconnections and interdependence, and the variety of forms these can take, as well as to realize that aging permeates everyone's life regardless of where we are in the life cycle–whether it be through the older people we know or through our own aging process. Aging is, after all, a lifelong process proceeding imperceptibly at every moment of our lives.

The *Strategies* were not invented out of whole cloth. An international consensus already exists about almost all of them–they have been drawn from a variety of action plans and declarations approved by conferences such as the 1995 World Summit for Social Development, the 1995 Beijing Conference on Women, the 1994 International Conference on Population and Development and, of course, the 1982 World Assembly on Aging. In the *Strategies*, these recommendations are simply reorganized into a different framework emphasizing life cycle, intergenerational, and society-wide perspectives (see Exhibit 1). As such, they may appeal to a broader audience that can identify personally with many of the provisions.

EXHIBIT 1

SELECTED STRATEGIES

1. **Among the key strategies that can be promoted by governments, businesses and unions, educational institutions, nongovernmental organizations, and other appropriate parties to assist individuals in moving
   successfully from one life stage to another are to:**

   (In the area of economic security)

   - Give both women and men full and equal access to economic resources,
     including the right to inheritance, the ownership of land and credit, as well
     as the opportunity to acquire their own rights in social security systems
     where they exist.

   (In the area of employment and other productive activity)

   - Promote a flexible approach to employment and productive activity, re-
     moving disincentives for part-time, temporary or volunteer work and facili-
     tating the continued employment of individuals regardless of age who
     have the desire and ability to extend their labor force participation.

   (In the area of education)

   - Provide affordable access to basic education, literacy training, vocational
     training, adult and other lifelong learning opportunities for all groups in so-
     ciety regardless of arbitrary characteristics such as age, gender, ethnicity,
     disability, or religion.

   (In the area of health)

   - Promote a healthy lifestyle, including education about lifestyle choices
     which contribute to healthy and long lives, such as decisions related to
     nutrition, exercise, and high risk behaviors involving tobacco, alcohol and
     drug use, and certain sexual practices.

2. **Among the key strategies that can be promoted by governments, businesses and unions, educational institutions, nongovernmental organizations, and other appropriate parties to support and strengthen intergenerational ties are to:**

   - Assist in keeping families and other social networks intact, including those
     of refugees and immigrants, while, at the same time, promoting tolerance
     for diverse family structures;
   - Facilitate multigenerational exchanges and collaboration in the pursuit of
     both personal and public interests, including mentoring relationships be-
     tween different age groups.

3. **Among the key strategies that can be promoted by governments, businesses and unions, educational institutions, nongovernmental organizations, and other appropriate parties to reduce tensions between individuals and society are to:**

- Provide the means through which individuals can influence decisions with major impact on their lives;
- Eliminate discriminatory practices that marginalize or exclude any group based on arbitrary characteristics such as age, gender, ethnicity, religion, or disability where they bear little or no relationship to performance in employment, volunteer roles and political life;
- Promote easier transitions throughout the lifespan between periods of education, work and leisure.

THE INTERDEPENDENCE OF LIFE STAGES

The first section of the *Strategies* examines the interdependence of life stages. An optimal old age–one in which human potential has been realized and "life has been added to years"–is not reached without considerable preparation in earlier stages of life for later physical, psychological, spiritual, and social well-being. Preparation at every life stage provides a platform for meeting the challenges of the next life stage. To become a psychologically mature person, one must be able to navigate all life stages, successfully coping with their responsibilities and problems. A life well-lived, in turn, can provide meaning, comfort, and satisfaction in the later years–qualities that can be shared with the generations that follow.

The growing likelihood everywhere of living to old age should and does influence choices in younger years. Individual self-reliance and foresight are required, but society can do much to provide the setting in which such virtues flourish.

This section is by far the longest, with 25 recommendations dealing with economic security, employment, education, health, environment and housing, and social services.

In the area of economic security, for example, it is recommended that both women and men have *the opportunity to acquire their own rights in social security systems where they exist.* This recommendation was included because poverty is more widespread among older women than older men almost everywhere in the world. Factors contributing to this phenomenon include women's more erratic participation in the labor force, with lengthy periods of "time out" because of caregiving responsibilities for both young and older family members. Wives' resulting dependence on husbands' pensions places divorced women at considerable risk in most countries with social security systems.

Countries such as Switzerland, Germany, and Canada have taken measures to address these quandaries. All three have introduced the notion of "pension splitting," in which marital partners' earnings during a marriage are pooled and divided equally for contribution and entitlement purposes. In case of divorce, the woman will share equally in what was jointly produced during the marriage. In both Switzerland and France, the primary child-rearing partner (usually the wife) is credited for years spent outside the labor force in raising children or caring for disabled persons. Such policies recognize the economic and social contributions made by women outside of the labor force in a very practical and meaningful way. They introduce more gender equity in the pension structure even if, for the time being in countries where overall pension levels are low, such policies do not immediately reduce poverty among older women.

In countries without well-developed social security systems, the importance of women having access to economic resources in old age, such as *the right to inheritance, the ownership of land and credit,* becomes even more critical. In some developed countries, for example, legal and customary barriers exist that prevent widows from inheriting land or women of any age from obtaining credit from banking institutions. Lending models such as the Grameen Bank in Bangladesh have shown that the availability of credit to women on easy terms results not only in flourishing microenterprises but in timely loan repayments.

THE INTERCONNECTEDNESS OF GENERATIONS

The second section of the *Strategies* looks at the rich interconnections that exist within and across age groups. No one is a member of just one group–age group or other; most of us participate in a number of communities of interest that transcend age divisions. Older people themselves do not view themselves as a separate group, but insist on remaining an integral part of society. A society without such interconnections probably could not survive.

The conflicts sometimes evident between members of different generations or even of the same generation can mask our common needs for love, emotional support, physical contact, respect and recognition; for the exchange of knowledge and experience; and for economic support and care. The extent of need will vary from individual to individual, from age group to age group, and from culture to culture. Each generation also stands on contributions made by earlier generations, instilling both respect for those who have gone before and a sense of stewardship towards future generations.

At the same time, each generation brings unique skills or qualities–the old are the only group that has lived through many of the experiences that younger generations have yet to encounter, and can serve as valuable role models.

Older persons may be carriers of unique cultures or traditions threatened with extinction or repositories of valuable skills, such as knowledge of traditional health practices. The young, in turn, bring a special energy and enthusiasm to life from which older and often more conservative temperaments can benefit. Some of their skills, such as knowledge of the latest technologies, can be very useful to older people. Different generations, by supporting one another, can strengthen both their societies and themselves.

Providing opportunities to and meeting the needs of different generations holds the potential for enhancing the lives of everyone. The view of such practices as constituting a "burden" ignores the rich web of interconnectedness in which we are all bound.

Thus, one of the recommended strategies is *to assist in keeping families and other social networks intact.* In many developing countries, extended families are being torn apart upon moving to urban areas because of lack of housing large enough to accommodate multiple generations. Constructive responses to this dilemma have been to give families that include a grandparent first choice in new public housing that becomes available or to permit extended families to tear down walls between adjacent apartments. Tax credits have also been extended to families that continue to provide support to an older family member.

THE INTERDEPENDENCE OF INDIVIDUALS AND SOCIETY

Finally, one cannot overlook the interdependence of individuals and the many social, religious, and political groups that represent them and the society in which they live. These groups intersect and interact constantly, sometimes harmoniously, sometimes in conflict. An examination of where tensions exist between individuals, or their organizational representatives, and the structures of society–tensions with potentially great impact on the quality of life of today's and tomorrow's older population–is required in moving towards a society for all ages.

An example from industrialized countries is the desire for easier and more frequent transitions between periods of education, work, and leisure than now exist, yet many societies are still rigidly structured in offering only sequential periods of education, work, and retirement.

While no society has achieved flexible life scheduling or even espouses it, in some post-industrial societies employers are becoming more responsive to the demands of their labor force by offering a variety of flexible work arrangements, such as compressed work schedules, part-time work, job splitting, sabbaticals, and educational leave. These options provide employees an opportunity to achieve a better balance between work, family life, education, and leisure. Interestingly, at the level of national policy, the notion of flexible life scheduling is reflected in the old age policies of countries such as Austria, Denmark, France, Germany, Luxembourg, Spain, and Sweden where gradual retirement is being encouraged through the offer of partial pensions. In principle, partial pensions permit older workers to either work longer or retire earlier (depending on one's perspective) by working part-time and drawing a partial pension for the work hours sacrificed. This option is also designed to facilitate a comfortable transition to full retirement.

The success of this policy has varied from country to country; it seems clear that comprehensive public policies are critical to its success. For example, social security systems in which pension benefits are based on earnings in the last five years of working life probably require modification if partial pensions are to be added. In addition, financial incentives for both employers and employees are recommended.

I might add that both the theme for the Year, as well as the proposed *Strategies*, have not met without controversy. There is a strong minority opinion in the United States and some European countries, which believes the selection of the theme "Towards a Society for All Ages" does a disservice to older persons. Instead, a continued emphasis on the special needs of older persons is urged before they are "mainstreamed" into the larger society. Similarly, the emphasis in the proposed *Strategies* on interdependence evokes an undesirable dependence for some. I might add that so far I have found no one in any developing country who has had such a reaction. On the contrary, respondents there cannot envisage a state in which older persons are considered in isolation from the rest of society.

CONCLUSION

As we move into a new century with ever greater numbers of older persons, it seems appropriate to rethink policy directions in dealing with this new demographic phenomenon. An approach that encourages the adaptation of key institutions to societal aging, and the preparation of persons of all ages for their eventual old age, while at the same time improving their current well-being, has obvious merit and may be better positioned to win public and policymakers' support than programs targeted to older persons alone. A framework for future policy direction along these lines is proposed in the document *Strategies for a Society for All Ages* as a supplement to key UN action plans, such as the Vienna International Plan of Action on Aging.

Depending on their stage of social and economic development, many countries may find that some of the strategies proposed carry great cost and are not viable from a practical point of view in the short range. Other strategies are less resource intensive but require a change in values or frames of thought. Some strategies can be introduced incrementally as part of more general legislative and regulatory reforms or institutional practices. Taken together, however, they outline some clear policy directions for the key actors in society.

NOTE

1. The complete *Strategies* is a policy document developed at AARP, an American nongovernmental organization representing older persons. The document was intended to provide meaning to the United Nations theme for the celebration of the International Year of Older Persons in 1999. It is available in English, French, and Spanish and can be viewed on the Internet at http://aarp.org/intl/strategies.html or at http://www.aoa.dhhs.gov/international/soc-allage-eng.html. For print copies, contact: International Activities, AARP, 601 E St., NW, Washington, DC 20049, USA.

The Elderly's Future Stake in Voluntary Associations

W. Andrew Achenbaum, PhD

University of Houston
Houston, Texas

KEYWORDS. Voluntary associations, social organizations, old-age interest groups

"There is only one country on the face of the earth where the citizens enjoy unlimited freedom of association for political purposes," observed Alexis de Tocqueville in *Democracy in America* (1835-40, p. 205). "This same country is the only one in the world where the continual exercise of the right of association has been introduced into civil life, and where all the advantages which civilization can confer are procured by means of it."

De Tocqueville's insights remain on target: A distinctive feature of American society from its founding to the present day has been the manner in which U.S. political organizations and civic institutions conjoin to promote individual success and to advance collective well-being. Such voluntary associations bind us in ways that governmental agencies do not. As urbanization, industrialization, and professionalization have transformed American society, voluntary associations have forged linkages between political and civic spheres. These arrangements generally have been more advantageous to white, native-

---

W. Andrew Achenbaum is Professor of History and Dean of the College of Humanities, Fine Arts, and Communication at the University of Houston. He chairs the board of directors of the National Council on Aging. He can be contacted care of the Office of the Dean, College of Humanities, Fine Arts, and Communication, University of Houston, Houston, TX 77204-3784 (E-mail: achenbaum@uh.edu).

[Haworth co-indexing entry note]: "The Elderly's Future Stake in Voluntary Associations." Achenbaum, W. Andrew. Co-published simultaneously in *Journal of Aging & Social Policy* (The Haworth Press, Inc.) Vol. 11, No. 2/3, 2000, pp. 41-47; and: *Advancing Aging Policy as the 21st Century Begins* (ed: Francis G. Caro, Robert Morris, and Jill R. Norton) The Haworth Press, Inc., 2000, pp. 41-47. Single or multiple copies of this article are available for a fee from The Haworth Document Delivery Service [1-800-342-9678, 9:00 a.m. - 5:00 p.m. (EST). E-mail address: getinfo@haworthpressinc.com].

41

born, middle-class males than to other segments of the population. Our national penchant for creating social organizations with political agendas in the 20th century has proven particularly beneficial to senior citizens.

This essay has three aims. It traces how old-age interest groups gained in visibility and power during the "modern" era. Next, it assesses what is called the "gray" lobby's current strengths and liabilities. The piece ends with speculations concerning the elderly's future stake in voluntary associations.

AGING INTEREST GROUPS ARE VOLUNTARY ASSOCIATIONS

According to de Tocqueville, the exercise of democracy in America has afforded U.S. citizens considerable opportunity and choice. Mobility-geographic, social, and economic–has sustained this felicitous situation for nearly four centuries. Americans of all ages have preferred to be on the go, freely deciding when to pull up stakes in their relentless search for fresh adventures. Each generation has found new frontiers to conquer, and seemingly boundless wealth to be gained. Confident of their Manifest Destiny, men and women in the new land have made self-reliance their most cherished virtue.

But despite grand hopes, even the most daring U.S. entrepreneurs have hedged their risks throughout our history. Out of enlightened self-interest, they created voluntary associations. Uncertainties in a new country, natural and otherwise, necessitated alliances among people who prefer to be their own masters. Americans made it a practice to be friendly to strangers, because they never knew when they might need a helping hand. Generations of farmers, laborers, and shopkeepers forged partnerships through voluntary associations. Seasoned landowners and aging manufacturers groomed successors for the day in which they would no longer be productive. The work ethic has deep roots here: Until the 1930s in the absence of Social Security, most cohorts of Americans labored hard all their lives, expecting at least modest rewards in due course.

U.S. politics has been as volatile as the booms and busts that have characterized our economy. Until relatively recently, local elections mattered more than national ones: property disputes, school taxes, road construction, and welfare burdens were considered parochial issues. Anyone with a legitimate stake in the community was encouraged to vote, but leaders were generally drawn from men of property, experience, and standing. At first, factions dominated government at all levels; in the 19th century, a two-party system took shape, each group claiming the vital center as its own. Politicians extolled voters' freedom of choice while appealing to their self-interest in domestic affairs.

No special institutions existed for older Americans in the early years of the Republic. We associate the tragedy of old-age dependency in the 19th century with the shadow of the poorhouse, but for most of its existence that dreaded institution served as the place of last resort for orphans, the handicapped, and the poor of any age. Retirement was not the norm before World War II. Families, religious groups, and local charities served young and old alike. Somehow they managed to provide access to whatever assistance "worthy" elders and children needed in order to subsist. Age was a less salient political factor than a citizen's race, gender, ethnicity, or drinking habits. There was one major exception: the Grand Army of the Republic (founded in Abraham Lincoln's hometown in 1866) was at once a fraternal order and a lobbying agency. With hundreds of thousands of members in Northern towns and cities, the G.A.R. secured from the U.S. Treasury more than $1 billion in benefits for Union soldiers and dependents by 1907. As Civil War survivors grew older, military pensions became the largest cash transfer available to citizens (Vinovskis, 1990).

Two historical trends are worth noting. On the one hand, the G.A.R. was not the nation's first voluntary association. Churches and synagogues, schools, political parties (not to mention the Sons and Daughters of the American Revolution) all targeted resources for children before they concentrated on senior citizens. But when veterans mobilized, they created a civic organization whose membership and effectiveness signified its political power–just as de Tocqueville observed. On the other hand, the G.A.R. did not view itself primarily as a vehicle for alleviating old-age dependency. Draped in patriotic glory, its officers stressed sacrifices once made on the battlefield. Advocates rarely mentioned that most of the intended beneficiaries happened to be old men and elderly widows. Hence, we must look to recent history for voluntary associations that benefit senior citizens in indirect ways as well as in a direct manner.

DOES THE GRAY LOBBY NOW ENJOY TOO MUCH FREEDOM OF ASSOCIATION?

The U.S. gray lobby has emerged as a network of voluntary associations that conform to patterns described in *Democracy in America.* It has grown enormously during the past 30 years in terms of size, variety, membership, and influence. There are more than a hundred national organizations that (1) provide services for older Americans or (2) advocate on behalf of elderly constituencies or (3) represent those professionals who work with the aged (Binstock & Day, 1996). The American Association for Retired Persons, which counts at least 37 million members over the age of 50 who are willing to pay $8 per year to receive discounts on prescription drugs and traveling among other benefits, is the second largest social organization in the United States after the Roman Catholic Church. Some agencies earmark subsets of the older population as their own, making it their *raison d'etre* to cater to particular ethnic, occupational, and regional constituencies. Other voluntary associations–such as religious bodies and alumni groups–create special niches for members of long standing. Various volunteer agencies (including political parties) seek out retirees: Those people with a history of giving of their time to others or for broader social purposes make especially attractive prospects.

Pluralistic purposes and diverse constituencies in the gray lobby rarely allow for a united front. Coalition building has been as essential as it has been for environmentalists, business roundtables, and welfare reformers. Hence, the National Council on the Aging consists of federated organizations; Generations United brings together groups representing different segments of the life course to broader social aims. Their *modus operandi* conforms to the style described by de Tocqueville (1956, p. 208) more than 150 years ago: "In these political associations, the Americans, of all conditions, minds, and ages, daily acquire a general taste for association. . . . They meet together in large numbers–they converse, they listen to each other, and they are mutually stimulated to all sorts of undertakings."

U.S. old-age interest groups have become major players in the policy arena. Through their efforts, the 1961 and 1971 White House Conferences on Aging set the stage for a series of legislative initiatives that liberalized Social Security coverage and benefits, established the first federal provisions for hospital insurance, and resulted in the creation of a wide range of social services, housing and transportation options, and employment opportunities for men and women over 65. No other nation in the world has relied so heavily on policy-oriented voluntary associations.

For all of the gray lobby's accomplishments, however, recent developments have not been auspicious. The Reagan Administration stifled the 1981 White House Conference on Aging; the 1995 gathering was so platitudinous as to call into question whether any visionary purpose was to be served by future conferences. Despite the health-care needs of a growing elderly population, Congress overturned the Medicare Catastrophic Coverage Act–in part because older Americans associated with the National Committee to Preserve Social Security and Medicare joined with AARP members (who had advocated for the measure) demanded such action. Because of competition for power and voice within its diverse constituencies, various segments of the gray lobby do not offer unequivocal support on how to reform long-term care. No wonder President Clinton, who could not marshall support for major medical reforms, has difficulty gaining support even for financing senior-citizen prescription medications. Meanwhile, the gray lobby has taken some nasty lumps. Americans for Generational Equity charged that paying for old-age entitlements was going to bankrupt youthful cohorts. Pundits in the 1980s began calling AARP loyalists "greedy geezers." Most old-age organizations seem more preoccupied with growing their membership rolls than preparing for the challenges and opportunities inherent in societal aging.

To place most of the blame for the current malaise in old-age policymaking on the gray lobby is unfair, of course. Many players with other agencies have contributed to the sorry state of affairs. The media has decided, and apparently its audience agrees, that increasing numbers of long-lived elders places a "growing burden" on resources. Federal reforms nowadays aim to reduce the elderly's entitlements, not expand them: Need-based initiatives are perceived as more efficient and less costly than benefits triggered to satisfy age-based criteria. Some philosophers have joined politicians in calling for a ceiling on health-care for the elderly on ethical as well as fiscal grounds. In this context, the gray lobby must adapt or be willing to lose ground.

LIKELY FUTURE SCENARIOS

Historians make better Monday-morning quarterbacks than long-term forecasters. Professionals who study the American experience that made up our national history, moreover, tend to highlight incremental changes rather than revolutionary developments; specialists generally concur that most transformative trends occur gradually. What follows, therefore, is a conservative assessment of how likely alterations in the elderly's stake in voluntary associations might affect old-age policymaking.

We begin with continuities, since they will predominate in the proximate future. The American Association for Retired Persons is bound to remain the largest and most influential U.S. organization for the elderly. Based on past and current operation, AARP can be expected to urge improvements in Social Security and innovations in health-care programs that will benefit millions of senior citizens. But AARP does not represent, and cannot speak for, all older Americans; the gray lobby will continue to be a mosaic. This nation, ever more pluralistic, will depend on many voices to advocate on behalf of its heterogeneous, ever-changing older population. Smaller groups may find it efficient to collaborate or merge. Coalition-building at both the federal and grassroots levels will remain the *sine qua non* of gray-lobby interactions.

Innovative institutional arrangements will flourish. A model will be Generations United, which provides a common meeting ground for those who advocate on behalf of children and youth and for those who represent the interests of the elderly. Elements of the gray lobby will reach out to other constituencies with whom they can forge mutually beneficial partnerships. Two such linkages, already under way, will probably grow in importance.

First, women's groups inevitably will see advantages in working with aging organizations. Not only are there more older women than older men but, historically, both groups have focused on the same set of gender-specific inequities. Women's financial concerns and medical priorities in later years have not been given the full attention that most policymakers know that they deserve. Focusing on women's issues provides a way of addressing needs-based policy goals that envelop class- or race-based disparities.

Second, I think that organizations representing the disabled and groups serving the elderly should continue to figure out ways to complement one another. This is a more debatable proposal than privileging feminist perspectives in gerontology. Most researchers and practitioners do not like to perpetuate notions that frailties color the experiences of late life. There are exceptions: Several editors of this journal have lobbied for "self direction" in home care for the disabled and the elderly. Gerontologists by and large prefer to work on changing images of old age as a disease. Similarly, those who speak on behalf of those with mental illness, back injuries, or AIDS prefer to carve out a clear-cut niche for themselves. Such definition makes it easier to solicit funds from specific sources; to embrace holistic perspectives on growing older, it is feared, can dilute the message. There is common ground, however: investigations into elderly people's chronic ailments are burgeoning. Specialists in public health, medical research, social science, and the humanities are collaborating in studies of arthritis, hearing loss, diabetes, and depression. In such domains experts can talk constructively about the potentialities manifest in people often marginalized.

More instantaneous, even serendipitous, associations can thrive in the Age of the Internet. Web sites for aging serve a useful purpose. When my 7-year-old niece was diagnosed with osteosarcoma, I was impressed by how much information I could retrieve by surfing the Web. And some of my fears, before surgery and during chemotherapy, were allayed by reading other people's comments on bulletin boards. I exchanged e-mails with strangers who knew how I felt. As more and more Americans become adept at using this technological treasure, voluntary associations may become virtual realities in which to voice concerns and mobilize support.

Most of us, of course, do not wish to reinvent ourselves each time that we log on. We muddle along as continuity theories of aging intimate. At midlife we are still sampling some of the same joys and losses of the heart we encountered earlier in life. Many Americans build their lives on enduring commitments: They rely on a few people–family, friends, and colleagues–with whom they interact over long periods of time. The shape of modern times thus fuels communitarian impulses in the United States. In an analogous way, old-age policymaking evolves slowly. Advances occur at the margins. Policymakers thus should monitor developments overseas, yet they should not expect other nations to adapt prototypes from our gray lobby. Nor are we likely to transplant foreign policies into native soil.

We should imagine our future selves in global terms, but we should capitalize on local environments. Established community-based resources–such as religious organizations and schools–are likely magnets for activities across generations. The family remains the first line of defense in times of need. And just as was the case in de Tocqueville's era, aging individuals are those best qualified to determine what is best for them–assuming that they have access to a variety of options in their immediate area. In the future as in the past, voluntary associations must provide citizens with structures that create such options, a forum to evaluate what exists, and a process that legitimates constructive improvements in the status quo.

REFERENCES

Binstock, R.H., & Day, C.L. (1996). Aging and politics. In R. H. Binstock and L. K. George (Eds.), *Handbook of aging and the social sciences*, 3rd ed. (pp. 362-87). San Diego: Academic Press.

de Tocqueville, Alexis (1835-40). In *Democracy in America* (Ed., Richard D. Heffner) (1956). York: Mentor, 1956.

Vinovskis, M.A. (Ed.) (1990). *Toward a social history of the American civil war.* New York: Cambridge University Press.

EMPLOYMENT AND RETIREMENT

Gradual Retirement in Europe

Genevieve Reday-Mulvey, MA

The Geneva Association
Geneva, Switzerland

KEYWORDS. Aging, work, retirement, transition, Europe

Flexibility in retirement is a crucial issue today and is destined to remain so for a number of reasons–the changing shape of pension schemes themselves and the end-of-career adjustments affecting enterprise and the workforce concerned.

Genevieve Reday-Mulvey is coordinator of the program on Work and Retirement, The Four Pillars, at the Geneva Association (International Association for the Study of Insurance Economics), launched in 1987 with the aim of proposing solutions to the challenge of population aging. She set up an international network on gradual retirement and, in 1996, edited the book *Gradual Retirement in the OECD Countries: Macro and Micro Issues and Policies*. She has prepared reports for the Swiss Federal Office of Social Affairs and for the European Commission and edits the twice-yearly research bulletin *The Four Pillars*. She can be contacted at the Geneva Association, 18 Ch. Rieu, CH-1208 Geneva (E-mail: geneva association@vtx.ch).

[Haworth co-indexing entry note]: "Gradual Retirement in Europe." Reday-Mulvey, Genevieve. Co-published simultaneously in *Journal of Aging & Social Policy* (The Haworth Press, Inc.) Vol. 11, No. 2/3, 2000, pp. 49-60; and: *Advancing Aging Policy as the 21st Century Begins* (ed: Francis G. Caro, Robert Morris, and Jill R. Norton) The Haworth Press, Inc., 2000, pp. 49-60. Single or multiple copies of this article are available for a fee from The Haworth Document Delivery Service [1-800-342-9678, 9:00 a.m. - 5:00 p.m. (EST). E-mail address: getinfo@haworthpressinc.com].

First, the future of pension systems. The issue of the current and future financing of state (i.e., "1st pillar") pensions[1] is already causing considerable concern in all European Union (EU) Member states as indeed in almost all Organization for Economic Cooperation and Development (OECD) countries. During the first half of the 1990s, demographic trends combined with pressure on public finances to bring about a radical change of direction in policymaking. The post-war "baby-boom" generation is now approaching retirement age (it will be reached between 2005 and 2010), and will be looking to its children and grandchildren, themselves members of a dwindling work force population, to provide for the comfortable pension package that has become the norm over the last 20 years. It is now common knowledge that the dependency ratio of nonactive retirees to active population is eroding rapidly and will have fallen from 1 to 5 in 1990 to just over 1 to 3 in 2020. Moreover, although most Member states of the EU have for economic as well as for social reasons encouraged early retirement over the last two decades, there has recently been a change in policy towards reversing this trend.

Most EU Member states have as a result undertaken substantial reforms which, in almost all cases, have involved building flexibility into the system at various points. At the same time, development of the 2nd pillar, already compulsory in certain countries like the Netherlands, the Nordic countries, France, and Switzerland, is being promoted by governments, and the financial foundation of this pillar (more often than not in the form of capitalization) is expected to make for greater flexibility in retirement in the future.

Second, flexible or gradual retirement is becoming increasingly relevant at the enterprise level. There is a growing awareness of the negative side of early-retirement policies. The loss of valuable expertise and corporate culture that early retirees take away with them into retirement is something that many firms could well do without. With the realization that sooner or later the problems of managing an aging work force will have to be addressed, the short-term nature of these early-retirement policies is becoming increasingly apparent. In any case, the required flexibility will be easier to achieve in today's world, which is rapidly developing new forms of employment (e.g., part-time work). The attitude of the trade unions is also beginning to change with the growing awareness that continuous training until end-of-career and adjusted conditions in the workplace are essential to the service-economy worker.

Third, flexible retirement is becoming a key issue also for the population at large whose life expectancy in good health (Morniche, 1996)[2] is rising steadily and who now wish to remain involved in the world of the workplace much later than hitherto. Such surveys as have been made reveal that most of the active population want greater flexibility as to the age of retirement and in the ways retirement is approached. Many qualified workers wish to work later, frequently with a change of work schedule and work station (e.g., working from home part of the time), and most would welcome a real transition between a full-time career and full retirement. The human life cycle itself is becoming increasingly supple, and it is essential that the occupational life cycle follows suite.

This article is in two parts:

- first, a brief account of recent trends in European legislation on public pensions as regards a more flexible and a later age of retirement;
- second, an analysis of the benefits and, of recent practice, of gradual retirement in three countries: France, Germany and Finland.

FLEXIBILITY AND RECENT PENSION REFORMS

The Influence of the European Commission

On December 10, 1982, the Council of the European Communities adopted a recommendation on the principles upon which a community policy on the age of retirement was to be based. Those principles were as follows:

- a loosening of the rules on the age of retirement, for example, flexibility making it possible to bring forward or defer the age of retirement;
- a gradual reduction in work time during the years preceding retirement;
- freedom to perform remunerated work for those already drawing an old-age pension.

In its report of July 2, 1986, the Commission proposed that over the next five years stress be laid on gradual retirement and on the cumulation of a pension and earned income. In its report of December 18, 1992, the Commission took stock of the reform process to date and concluded that most Member states through the introduction of reforms had brought national legislation into line with the principles of the 1982 Recommendation.

In May 1999 (COM 1999, 221 final) the Commission, in its communication *Towards a Europe for all Ages,* planned with the help of Member states "to identify ways and means of reversing the trend towards early retirement, to study new patterns of gradual retirement and to increase the viability and flexibility of pension schemes." In addition, the Commission invited Member States "to promote life-long training and flexible work patterns."

Main Features of Recent State Pension Reforms

There are basically six features of recent state pension reforms: (1) a rise in the age of retirement; (2) greater flexibility in the age of retirement and promotion of gradual retirement; (3) promotion of a lengthening of the contribution period and the freedom to combine a pension with income from work; (4) a curtailing of early retirement; (5) a reduction in the benefit level; and (6) changes in the way retirement is funded. Two of the measures in this list focus on flexibility.

Greater flexibility in the age of retirement and promotion of gradual retirement. In the Nordic countries (Sweden, Finland, Denmark, and Norway), save for Finland, retirement is entered into at a relatively late age, although the latter was lowered slightly under pressure from the economic recession of the early 1990s. In addition to the universal pension, in part financed from taxes, a supplementary pension is compulsory and, following the recent reforms, is now increasingly capitalization-based. A feature of these supplementary pensions, for which an extension of the contribution period is being encouraged, is their flexibility. In Sweden, the age of entitlement to the basic pension (for residents)[3] is 65 years old but, with the supplementary pension, there exists no upper age limit and employees increase their pension by working as late as possible. Wide use is made of flexible practice in order to be able to foster employment of workers at the end of their careers. Indeed, there exists a partial pension scheme for those 60 years old (about to be raised to 61) and older, whereby employees can work part-time and draw a partial pension. This scheme was introduced in 1976 and has proven to be very popular (especially in years when the partial-pension level has been high). Unfortunately, the conditions of this scheme will change in the year 2000 and be less generous. Older workers will be able to continue working part-time (there is no shortage of vacancies) but there will be no automatic payment of a partial pension.

- In Denmark, the reform of January 1995 was designed to promote gradual retirement by replacing the system of full early retirement with a part-time work regime. These measures concern wage earners between 60 and 65 old years who have been members of an unemployment insurance fund for at least 20 out of the last 25 years. Work time has to be reduced by at least one quarter. For the self-employed, work time must be reduced by 18.5 hours per week. A partial pension makes up the income gap. The deferment of retirement is encouraged also by the supplementary pension (there is an increase of 5% every six months within a overall ceiling of 30%).
- In Finland, a partial retirement scheme for wage earners 60 years old and older was introduced in both the private and public sectors in the late 1980s. To promote it, it was decided in the 1990s (1994 and 1997) to extend it to persons 56 years old and older and to provide a series of incentives (e.g., tax breaks for firms). Beneficiaries draw a part-time

wage supplemented by a partial pension which makes up 50% of the loss of earnings.

- In 1991, Belgium became one of the first countries to adopt flexible retirement between 60 and 65 years.
- In 1995, Italy opted for a flexible age of retirement between 57 and 65 years. Radical reform of the system in Italy will mean then hence forward a link will be established between benefit and contribution levels.
- In Germany, Austria, and France, there now exists the option to enter gradual or partial retirement before or after the retirement age. Other countries, like Spain and Luxembourg, have also built a little flexibility into their systems.

Promotion of a lengthening of the contribution period and freedom to combine a pension with income from work. Most of the recent reforms are designed to encourage a longer contribution period by making the amount of the pension directly dependent on the length of contribution. This applies more particularly to recent reforms in Italy (1995) and Sweden (1994), and also to some extent to Finland, the United Kingdom, Denmark, and Germany.

With the exception of Spain, all EU Member states now allow the cumulation of a pension and income from work. Some countries have set a ceiling on income from work (Italy, Belgium, Denmark, and Greece) or have special conditions (France).

GRADUAL RETIREMENT IN EUROPE

Benefits of Gradual Retirement

Gradual retirement, also known as phased, partial, or part-time retirement, provides a transition period between a full-time career and complete cessation of paid work. The worker, instead of working full time one day and fully retiring the next, can reduce work hours according to graduated and agreed schedules while drawing part-time pay and, in some cases, some form of partial pension. Many formulae for workload downsizing exist, and the transition periods during which this occurs can run for anywhere from 1 to 10 years. Approximately five years is the transition period most commonly encountered in the OECD countries, while in recent legislation in France and Germany, work-time reduction is planned for workers between 55 and 65. Gradual retirement can be used to reduce working life as well as to extend it. In Sweden, gradual retirement, was originally designed to facilitate a shortening of working life. However, in countries like France, Germany, Austria, Finland, and Denmark, current government policy is to exert pressure in order to reverse the trend towards early retirement, and gradual retirement is being used as a replacement for full early retirement.

There are a number of advantages for employers and workers alike.

For the employer, gradual retirement or work-time reduction:

- reduces the wage-cost of hours worked;
- raises productivity per hour (productivity per hour in many work functions increases when a worker moves from full- to part-time);
- helps retain within the firm skills and expertise together with the older worker's specific contribution;
- reduces absenteeism generally high at the end of the career (e.g., Swedish and French firms);
- increases job satisfaction whenever the firm is in a position to retain the older employee in interesting work and conserve the latter's social benefits; and
- makes for better age management (filling vacated work-time with younger employees as in French firms); frees older workers for training duties.

For the employee, gradual retirement or work-time reduction:

- makes it possible to adapt work to the older worker's changing abilities;
- reduces stress and increases job satisfaction;
- gives the older worker the opportunity to benefit from continued membership in a work team and from inclusion in the workplace (e.g., Japan); and
- provides the older worker with free time to develop extra-occupational activities.

Our research over the last few years has revealed that gradual retirement can constitute an excellent and very flexible mode for end-of-career management and that its potential for a flexible extension of working life is considerable in most OECD countries. When properly prepared for at the enterprise and individual levels, it can, in the short term, provide a bridge between the currently receding official age for retirement and today's all-too-early effective age of exit from the workforce. It offers a halfway house between employee and employer and an opportunity, in some cases with state support, for a sharing of the cost of this stage in the life cycle. In the longer term, it is, we believe, destined to become the standard mode for extension of working life beyond any notional or reference retirement age. It could reduce the future costs of retirement pensions by allowing a partial pension which tops up the earnings of workers, or part-time retirees (hence the term "the 4th pillar"), rather than having to grant a full pension.

Implementation of Gradual Retirement
in France, Germany, and Finland

Recent studies show that extension of working life is seen everywhere as a crucial policy for reducing the future burden of social expenditure. Because of its flexible nature, which is well suited to end of career, gradual retirement is finding increasing favor with the majority of workers, and growing acceptance with management and trade unions. In our book *Gradual Retirement in the OECD Countries, Macro and Micro Issues and Policies*, a typology of four models was proposed: the Swedish, Japanese, Continental, and Anglo-Saxon models. We have space here to cite only the recent experience in France, Germany, and Finland. However, it is important to remember that Sweden has been the country where gradual retirement has developed most over the last two decades–in the early 1990s, about a third of workers between 60 and 65 were in gradual retirement while benefitting from a partial pension. The reasons for its success in Sweden were availability of part-time jobs, a good partnership between government and employers, and the high replacement rate of partial pensions.

Due to financial constraints, reforms to the pension system were introduced in June 1994 by removing the partial pension, which made gradual retirement much less attractive. Finland and Denmark are following the Swedish model of the last two decades by promoting gradual retirement combined with a partial pension, while France and Germany promote gradual retirement before the age of retirement through financial incentives to firms (which supplement part-time income) with a view to reversing the trend towards early retirement. It is only after the age of retirement that a partial pension is made available for workers continuing part-time.

France, Germany, Finland, and other continental European countries have been characterized by a practice of very early retirement which has been encouraged over the last two decades by public policies. It is true that labor-force participation rates in these countries have reflected more the availability of generous social-security provision than the situation of labor markets. Over recent years, disability, unemployment and early retirement routes–"loopholes for those who want to retire" (Schmähl et al., 1994) have been reduced significantly, but they will have to be made even less accessible and more expensive in the future.

In *France*, since the early 1990s, but especially since 1993, government policy has attempted to reverse the early retirement trend. By providing subsidies and incentives, gradual early retirement has developed well over the last five years. Partial early retirement is designed essentially for voluntary employees from 55 to 65 years. The employee earns a wage paid by the employer for the part-time hours he or she has worked and, until retirement, receives for the unworked half-time a supplement equal to about 30% (pro-

vided the firm fills the vacated time with new employees) of the daily reference wage (up to a ceiling). The income is evenly spread over the entire
period even in cases where the half-time is worked on a pluri-annual basis.
This scheme has the approval of both employer representatives and the
unions. Business leaders view the scheme as an opportunity for off-loading
certain categories of employee, for rejuvenating the age profile of their work
force, for developing part-time positions throughout their staff structure and
for improved management of work-force skills. The unions and workers see
it as a way of reducing work hours on favorable financial and occupational
terms for flagging employees approaching the end of their careers. Even so,
gradual retirement is still frequently perceived as "second best" by comparison with early retirement, which certain firms and certain sectors in difficulty
have continued to enjoy.

By the end of 1998, partial early retirement involved over 80,000 private-
sector workers benefitting from state-subsidized schemes. Finns in all sectors
and of all sizes (hospitals, building, manufacturing, services, banking and
insurance) have been involved. Examples of firms having adopted gradual
retirement schemes are: in the manufacturing sector, Rhône-Poulenc, Aéro-
spatiale, Total, Framatome, Elf Atochem, Péchiney Emballage Alimentaire,
Péchiney Rhénalu, IBM, Hewlett-Packard; in services, Crédit Agricole, Casi-
no, AXA, UAP, and many hospitals. Even if this number represents less than
10% of the workers concerned, it indicates the future direction of policies and
practice. In September 1999, a report was prepared for Prime Minister, Mr.
Jospin, on policies for promoting gradual retirement.

Gradual retirement also facilitates skills transfer and the supervision of
newcomers to the work force to fill the works hours vacated by part-time
gradual retirees–"traineeship schemes" is the name given to such supervised
apprenticeship arrangements, most frequently encountered in industry and
construction.

In *Germany*, one of the key features of the law, which came into force on
August 1, 1996, is the promotion of part-time work for older workers, providing incentives for both employers and employees (providing the latter reduce
their work hours by half on reaching 55 years). Where the employer is
prepared to top up the employee's part-time earnings by 20% and pension
insurance contributions to a level corresponding to 90% of full-time pay, the
employer will, subject to certain conditions, be compensated for these payments by the Federal Labor Office. Collective agreements (VW, DB, Luf-
thansa, Preussen Elektra) have improved upon statutory requirements. In
these companies, the employees get 85% of their last salary for working half
time. Collective agreements exist now in a number of branches–the chemical
industry, the power plant sector, insurance, and elsewhere. At the end of
1998, over 30,000 workers were on some form of gradual retirement, and the

government is due to propose accompanying measures to encourage its development.

In *Finland*, a partial retirement scheme for wage-earners 60 years old and older was introduced in the private sector in 1987 and in the public sector in 1989. The scheme, however, failed to attract many takers and more recently it was decided to extend it to persons 56 years old and older and to provide a series of incentives (e.g., tax breaks for Finns). Beneficiaries draw a part-time wage supplemented by a partial pension, which makes up 50% of the loss of earnings. For the time being, the main obstacle facing the scheme is the fact that, in contrast to other Nordic countries, there is a shortage of suitable part-time vacancies. Nevertheless, the future prospects for this partial pension scheme look encouraging and, in 1998, 11,000 workers were a part of it compared to 7,000 the previous year.

In these three countries, as is also the case in Sweden, the older workers taking up this part-time option must pledge in writing that they will not take up other professional commitments and, indeed, there is evidence that they do not. Therefore, they experience a real reduction of work time and a true transition between full-time work and complete retirement.

Recommendations for Public and Company Policies

Public policies. What stands out as essential is that public policies need to be sufficiently comprehensive and accompanied by incentives at various levels. Those countries that so far have been more successful in implementing gradual retirement tend to be the ones which have designed global policies (Sweden and Japan). It is essential to make early retirement options as well as disability and unemployment routes more difficult, more costly, and their terms more stringent. An objection will be made that current labor-market conditions, and especially high rates of unemployment, make any progress in the desired direction at this time very difficult. It is precisely for this reason that gradual retirement cannot be handled outside the broader context of employment redesign and redistribution. In several countries, recent legislation (or, in the Netherlands, collective agreements) is beginning to promote replacement of *full* early retirement with *gradual* early retirement, and to make retirement more flexible and occur later. But such legislation clearly needs to be accompanied by financial incentives from the state. The age at which gradual retirement can commence is also crucially important. Changing the deeply rooted mind-sets of the early retirement culture requires drastic redesign, a good partnership between the state and business, new age management policies, and their gradual implementation.

Company policies. Four areas at least, among the many that require attention, should be a particular focus for this integrated policy approach. The first area is training. In order for older workers to remain motivated and productive, continuing training should not terminate at 45 or 50 years old but should continue until the end of one's career. Countries in which such company policies exist are in a much stronger position when the decision to extend working life is made. In Sweden, the extent of training is impressive, and there seems to be very little discrimination towards older workers (Wadensjo, 1996). In France, especially in bigger companies, the same policy is to be found (Reday-Mulvey, 1994).

A second key variable is pay policy. It is now perfectly clear that seniority-based pay policy, by raising the wage costs of workers at end of career, constitutes a real obstacle to all forms of extension of working life. In several countries, there is a growing trend in wage calculation today towards reducing the weight of the seniority factor and increasing that of performance. In America and Britain, this trend is prevalent in bigger firms, but is now to be found in other countries (e.g., in Japan, Germany and France in some sectors, such as insurance).

Third is occupational pensions. Many Dutch, British, and American pension funds are final-salary based but there is an increasing consensus to modify them and make them average-salary based.

And the fourth area is part-time and flexible work. The development of part-time and flexible forms of employment is obviously important for gradual retirement. Most countries have seen such development at either end of the life cycle. Countries such as the Netherlands and the United Kingdom have a high rate of part-timers. Some have improved legislation in this respect so as to provide better levels of protection for part-time work (for example, France and the Netherlands). In other countries, there is availability of part-time jobs for older workers either inside (e.g., Sweden) or outside their main career employment (e.g., Japan, the United States, and the United Kingdom), but social protection for part-time employment has to be improved in the latter cases.

A FINAL WORD

Gradual retirement seems to stand at the crossroads of two important issues:

- redesigning the end of career and flexibly extending working life for pressing financial reasons, which have to do with demographic prospects, but also because of the need for proper management of human resources and skills; and
- developing well-protected and regular part-time and flexible work not only as a desirable transition from full employment to full retirement, but also as an ideal opportunity for moving towards a socially fairer and more efficient division of labor within our society (Giarini & Liedtke, 1997).

NOTES

1. The first pillar is the compulsory state pension, based on the pay-as-you-go principle; the second pillar is the supplementary occupational pension, normally based on funding; the third pillar is made up of individual savings (personal pensions, personal assets, and life insurance); and the fourth pillar is income from part-time work for some years after reaching retirement age, or sooner, in the case of early retirement.

2. In France, in the decade 1981-1990, life expectancy in good health increased by 3 years for men and 2.6 for women.

3. The basic pension is the social security pension, while the supplementary pension is the employer's pension.

REFERENCES

Bass, S.A., Caro, F.G., & Chen, Y.P. (Eds.) (1994). *Achieving a productive aging society,* Westport, CT/London: Auburn House.

Delsen, L., & Reday-Mulvey, G. (Eds.) (1996). *Gradual retirement in the OECD countries.* Aldershot, UK: Dartmouth.

Gaullier, X. (1993). *Salariés âgés: Conditions de travail et transition vers la retraite.* Rapport sur la France pour le Bureau International du Travail. Geneva: International Labour Office.

Giarini, O., & Liedtke, P. (1997). *The employment dilemma–The future of work.* Report for the Club of Rome, Geneva: International Association for the Study of Insurance Economics.

International Association for the Study of Insurance Economics. (1987-1999). *The Four Pillars Research Bulletin*, Nos. 4-25. Geneva: Author.

International Association for the Study of Insurance Economics. (1994, 1996, 1999). *The Geneva Papers on Insurance, Studies on the Four Pillars.* Geneva: Author.

Kohli, M., Rein, M., Guillemard, A., & van Gunsteren, H. (Eds.). (1991). *Time for retirement. Comparative studies of early exit from the labor force.* Cambridge: Cambridge University Press.

Kuhn, K., Lunde, A., Mirabile, M.L., Reday-Mulvey, G., & Taylor, P. (1998). *Career planning and employment of older workers.* Report for the European Commission, Maastricht, Driekant.

Morniche, P. (1996, April-June). Vie et sante progressent de concert. *Risques, Les Cahiers de l'Assurance, 26,* 21-22. Paris.

Naegele, G. (1999). Gradual retirement in Germany. *Journal of Aging & Social Policy, 10*(3), 83-102.

Reday-Mulvey, G. (1994, October). Continuing training until end of career. *The Geneva Papers on Risk and Insurance.* Geneva.

Schmähl, W., & Gatter, J. (1994). Options for extending the working period and flexibilizing the transition to retirement in the German insurance industry–The current situation and assessment for the future. *The Geneva Papers on Risk and Insurance, 1973,* 433-471.

Shimowada, I. (1992). Aging and the Four Pillars in Japan. *The Geneva Papers on Risk and Insurance, 17*(62), 40-80.

Takala, M. (1999). Part-time pensions in Finland. Paper presented at a conference "Active Strategies for an Ageing Workforce" in Turku, Finland, August 11-13, 1999. Helsinki: Central Pension Institute.

Takayama, N. (1998). The morning after in Japan: Its declining population, too generous pensions, and a weakened economy. Tokyo: Maruzen.

Wadensjo, E. (1996). Gradual retirement in Sweden. In L. Delsen and G. Reday-Mulvey (Eds.), *Gradual retirement in the OECD countries*. Aldershot, UK: Dartmouth.

Walker, A. (Ed.) (1994). *Older people in Europe-Social and economic policies: Recent developments*. Brussels: Commission of the European Communities.

Worsley, R. (1996). *Age and employment-Why employers should think again about older workers*. London: Age Concern.

Increasing Life Expectancy, Retirement Age, and Pension Reform in the German Context

Winfried Schmähl, Dr. rer. pol.

University of Bremen

KEYWORDS. Retirement age, pension reform, life expectancy, pay-as-you-go financing, German pension policy

In many industrialized countries, a rising percentage of the elderly in the population is often seen as an important challenge to the economy and to society because of the aging of "baby boomers"; smaller, younger cohorts, due to reduced fertility rates; and increasing life expectancy, especially of the elderly. In public debate, aging mainly is seen as a problem: discussion focuses on costs rather than benefits. The impact of aging populations on social security–pension schemes, health care, and long-term care insurance– is a major topic of political and scientific discussion in many countries. "Can we afford to grow older?" is an often-used phrase (Aaron, Bosworth, & Burtless, 1989; Bovenberg & van der Linden, 1997; Disney, 1996). Political proposals and decisions in many countries are aiming at a reduction of future expenditure development, especially in regard to public pension schemes.

Prof. Dr. Winfried Schmähl is Professor of Economics at the Centre for Social Policy Research at the University of Bremen, Bremen, Germany. He is also Chairman of the Social Advisory Board on Pension Policy to the German Federal Government. His research interests are social security, the effects of demographic aging, and pension policy. He can be contacted care of the Centre for Social Policy Research, University of Bremen, Parkallee 39, D-28209 Bremen, Germany (E-mail: schmaehl@zes.uni-bremen.de).

[Haworth co-indexing entry note]: "Increasing Life Expectancy, Retirement Age, and Pension Reform in the German Context." Schmähl, Winfried. Co-published simultaneously in *Journal of Aging & Social Policy* (The Haworth Press, Inc.) Vol. 11, No. 2/3, 2000, pp. 61-70; and: *Advancing Aging Policy as the 21st Century Begins* (ed: Francis G. Caro, Robert Morris, and Jill R. Norton) The Haworth Press, Inc., 2000, pp. 61-70. Single or multiple copies of this article are available for a fee from The Haworth Document Delivery Service [1-800-342-9678, 9:00 a.m. - 5:00 p.m. (EST). E-mail address: getinfo@haworthpressinc.com].

Time spent in retirement has not only increased in absolute terms, but is also relative to the whole life span as compared to the working life. It is argued that retirement ages are of central importance when trying to cope with the effects of increasing life expectancy on pension financing. That theme will be exemplified in the German context in this commentary, outlining some demographic trends, political approaches for dealing with future pension financing, and comparing them to alternative options. The discussion will be restricted to the effects of increasing life expectancy on pay-as-you-go financed public pension schemes. A special focus will be on measures directly linking life expectancy to certain elements of pension schemes.

AGING IN GERMANY

One of the indicators most often used to describe the aging of the population in a social policy context is the old-age dependency ratio (ADR), comparing the number of "elderly" to the number of persons in their "working life." Obviously, the definition depends on a decision as to when working life usually (or, on the average) starts, and when it ends. For international comparisons, an identical definition for all countries is useful; however, it often does not describe the conditions in a specific country.

Within the OECD countries as well as in Europe, Germany has one of the highest old-age dependency ratios. Defining ADR as persons aged 60 and older in relation to those between 15 and 59, in 1997, the average of all OECD countries was 18.9; of the countries of the European Union, 23.4; of Germany, 23.9 (OECD, 1999).

Taking into account the extended phase of education as well as the lowering of the effective retirement age, in Germany, a definition of ADR based on a working phase between 20 (not 15) and 59 is usually considered as relevant. The results of the most recent official population projection for Germany (based on only modest numbers of migrants, a continuous low fertility rate but a further increase of life expectancy)[1] give the following ADR figures: 1995, 35.8; 2010, 44.8; 2030, 73.2, and 2040, 76.4.

If, however, for example, up to 2040 an upward shift in the beginning of "old age" from 60 to 65 is assumed, the so-defined ADR would be "only" 56 instead of 76. But, as already mentioned, whether this can become a realistic assumption, and not only an artificial calculation, is–among other things–considerably linked to labor market conditions.

Since the early 1970s, male labor-force participation rates (LFPR) beyond age 55 have dropped drastically. One reason, however, not the only one, was the introduction of a "flexible" retirement age. Since 1973, it has become possible to claim a full pension (without deductions) as early as age 63 (women and the unemployed could claim the pension without deductions at age 60). To give an illustrative example: In 1970, LFPR of men age 63 was 67%. After the introduction of the flexible retirement age, LFPR dropped within two years to 47%, within 10 years to 27%, and now is around 20%. Regarding early retirement, there were "push" factors (labor-market conditions worsened) and "pull" factors (pre-retirement possibilities outside the public pension scheme were created).[2] Not only did the effective retirement age go down, but also the expectations of employees were focused on early retirement, and the age an employee became an "older" employee started earlier as well, reducing the chances to become re-employed after a period of unemployment. Over the years, early retirement became a well-accepted measure in Germany to cope with labor-market problems (before and after German unification) and to reduce the staff of firms.[3]

This was one important factor for extending the phase of retirement. The other factor was the increase in life expectancy, especially due to a reduction of mortality in higher adult age. For example, from 1960 up to 1995, life expectancy at age 65 increased relatively much faster than (average) life expectancy at birth. This increase in life expectancy during the last decades was much faster than in the previous period, from the turn of the century. In West Germany, around 1960, the life expectancy for women aged 65 was 79.6 years on average, i.e., a remaining life expectancy of 14.6 years. It increased by four years up to the mid-1990s (to 83.6 years). The difference in life expectancy of men and women aged 65 increased also during this period: About 1960, it was 2.2 years, and by the middle of the 1990s, it had become 3.8 years (i.e., 79.9 years for men). Both developments–higher life expectancy as well as a growing gap in male and female life expectancy–affect the financing of pension schemes because of an extended period of pension payment for the insured as well as for the surviving spouse (in general, the women).

In the official population projections in Germany, a further increase in life expectancy for the elderly is assumed also for the future.[4] These assumptions are mainly based on the fact that in some other industrialized countries higher life expectancies already exist. This can be illustrated by a new population projection which the German Central Statistical Office is now preparing (publication is expected at the end of 1999). In 1995, (remaining) life expectancy in Germany for those aged 60 was 18.1 years (for men) and 22.5 years (for women), while life expectancy, for example, in Japan and Switzerland was about two years higher (for men) and in Japan nearly three years higher for women. German forecasters are basing their assumptions on such facts and are assuming for the year 2035 an increase in life expectancy for men at age 60 of 2.5 years (to 20.6 years) and for women of 3.3 years (to 25.8 years).

LONGEVITY AND PENSION SCHEMES

Taking these tendencies into consideration, it becomes even more obvious that the division of the life cycle between working span and years in retirement shifts more and more towards the latter, if effective retirement ages remain more or less constant or even become lower over time. Additional years in retirement raise, *ceteris paribus*, the number of pensioners as well as the ratio of the number of pensioners to contributors. This pensioner ratio (systemic dependency ratio)[5] is one of the central determinants for contribution and/or tax rates to balance the budget of a pay-as-you-go (PAYG) financed pension scheme. Such a scheme is the statutory pension insurance (social insurance) plan in Germany. It is by far the largest scheme for old-age provision in Germany, with 70% of all expenditures for old-age security and more than 10% of GDP.[6]

The second decisive factor in a PAYG scheme is the (average) pension level, defined as the ratio of average pension benefits to average gross wages. In Germany–as in many countries–wages are the main source of social insurance contribution revenue.

An increase in life expectancy *ceteris paribus* makes old-age security more costly in a PAYG as well as in a (fully) capital-funded scheme.[7] In a PAYG scheme, contribution revenue has to be increased–by increasing the assessment base or by a higher contribution rate–or money from the state budget has to be transferred to the pension scheme. All these alternatives are, at least at present, difficult to realize politically. Especially in Germany, it is a much supported goal (politically) not to increase contribution rates and to avoid, via employers' contributions, an increase in labor costs because of intensified international competitiveness and expected negative effects for national labor markets.[8] The question, therefore, is how to react to the challenges arising from an aging of the population as well as from an aging of the labor force.

OPTIONS FOR REACTIONS

There are many possible ways to influence the number of retirees and contributors, the (average) pension benefit and (average) contributory wages, by instruments within the pension scheme or, for example, by tax incentives or economic policy measures.[9] In the following, I will focus on those measures within a public PAYG-financed pension scheme that directly links measures to life expectancy. Here, new developments can be seen that may receive more attention in the future.

If the (discounted) sum of pension benefits over the lifetime of an individual pensioner or of a cohort is to remain constant in the case of rising life expectancy, the annual pension benefits will have to be reduced, but benefits are paid out over a longer period. A reduction in the pension level becomes necessary if the pension benefit is started at an unchanged retirement age. An equivalent alternative concerning present value of accumulated pension benefits is to increase the age at which the pensioner is eligible for a pension, or–to be more precise–the age at which a full pension (without reductions) can be claimed. If the pension is claimed earlier, the (monthly) pension benefit is reduced to take into account longer duration of the pension.

In Sweden as well as in Latvia, and now also in Poland, the reform of the public pension scheme follows this line by introducing a defined contribution scheme: The accumulated nominal individual contribution payments of the insured person (including some imputed "interest") are transformed into an annuity by explicitly taking into consideration (remaining) life expectancy of the respective cohort. If life expectancy increases, a "younger" pensioner with identical accumulated pension claims receives a lower regular (monthly) pension benefit at a certain retirement age, compared to pensioners who retired earlier. This can be looked upon as an implicit measure for increasing retirement age.

A quite different approach was decided on by the German government in 1997: An additional factor was to be introduced into the pension formula resulting in a general reduction of the pension level for all pensioners (old and new) in case of increasing life expectancy (Schmähl, 1997, for details). After the election of the German Federal Parliament in autumn 1998, this measure was suspended (and will be abolished in the near future).

Today, the development of individual pension benefits over time in Germany's statutory pension scheme is linked to the growth rate of average net earnings, resulting in a constant ratio of (individual) pensions to average net earnings (net pension level). The additional factor (based on the development of life expectancy) would reduce the pension adjustment rate in case of increasing life expectancy, and therefore would reduce the net pension level for all current and future pensioners.[10]

A third approach for coping with the financial problems of higher life expectancy is linked to the definition of the "normal" retirement age, that is, the age for taking the full (unreduced) pension. An increase in life expectancy provides the chance for a reallocation of time in the life cycle by extending working life and not extending the time spent in retirement to the full amount of the increase in life expectancy.[11] Extending retirement ages and reducing earlier retirement is a topic now on the political agenda in many countries. However, as long as labor market conditions remain unfavorable–as they are at present in Germany–a conflict exists between short- and medium-term labor market requirements and long-term labor market as well as social political tasks. In 1992 and 1996, it was decided to phase in deductions from the full pension, aiming at a higher effective retirement age and reducing expenditure of the pension schemes. But unemployment is still high in Germany. Therefore, at the end of the century, government as well as some trade unions are aiming at a low effective retirement age by compensating for the deductions, arguing that this will improve one's chances to be integrated into the labor market, especially for young people. This assumption is, however, hardly based on empirical facts, at least for Germany. In the German political arena, the topic of increasing retirement ages in the future is being given no attention at present. Nevertheless, it remains an important issue to bring into this debate.

Increasing the effective retirement age does not only depend on changes in legal retirement ages in the public scheme but also on the design of occupational pension schemes, on labor-market conditions, health conditions[12] and especially on income from different sources (including income from work as well as from transfer payments, occupational pensions, and private saving) as well as on preferences of the individuals. Besides such ad hoc increase of "normal" (as well as earliest) retirement ages, a rule could be designed based on life expectancy development. Such a rule was proposed by the author for Germany (Schmähl, 1997, 1998a) as an alternative approach to the general reduction of the pension level the former government was aimed at. Such a rule can be announced some years before it becomes effective, giving employees as well as employers a chance to adapt to the new conditions. Increasing legal retirement ages can be based on an ad hoc decision.

The increase in "normal" (as well as earliest) retirement age will then follow the development of life expectancy with a time lag of several years. The increase in retirement ages, however, will be less than the increase in life expectancy–this will be shared between additional time in working life and retirement. To give an illustration of how to share an additional year of life expectancy, we assume that the (average) pension level is 0.5, the pensioner ratio 0.4 and therefore (no other revenue besides contributions), the contribution rate is 0.2. If life expectancy increases, the pensioner ratio would go up, if (effective) retirement ages remain constant. If the pensioner ratio is to remain at 0.4, 12 months of additional life expectancy "require" a higher retirement age (normal as well as earliest) of about 8.6 months. Therefore, additional time in retirement will increase, too, but "only" to 3.4 months.

Aaron and Reischauer (1998, p. 101) proposed a different rule for the United States after phasing in of the "normal" retirement age from 65 to 67 in the year 2011[13]: "Workers who spend the same portion of their lives in retirement as those terming at 62 in 2011 would receive unchanged benefits. In other words, if retirement should represent one fourth of adults in 2011, a one-year increase in adult longevity would lead to the benefit cut associated with a nine-month increase in the age at which unreduced benefits are paid."

Retiring prior to the increased "normal" retirement age results in a lower pension because of deductions from the full pension. The fundamental problem in decisionmaking is obvious: Work longer and receive the full pension or retire earlier with lower benefits. How workers (and their employers) will react to these new conditions depends on a great number of influencing factors. Workers can save to bridge the time span between exit from work and taking up the (public) pension. This can also result from occupational pension schemes or from (long-term) time-saving accounts.

Implementing such a strategy requires, however, several preconditions. One was already mentioned: Labor-market conditions should allow older workers to remain employed longer than they are today. For Germany, a remarkable reduction in labor supply is forecasted because of structural demographic changes.[14] Retraining of older workers becomes especially important from a microeconomic as well as macroeconomic point of view in order to increase or at least stabilize (age-specific) productivity. Instead of still offering incentives to retire earlier (as currently often proposed in Germany), incentives for human capital investments for older workers also seem to be an adequate public response to challenges ahead.

Investment in human capital even for older adults becomes more attractive for employees as well as employers, if the time for using human capital is extended (because of older retirement ages). Here, the interaction between social policy regulations, decisions by employees and employers, and labor-market conditions becomes obvious. It also underlines the necessity of comprehensive analysis as well as comprehensive approaches in preparing political decisions.

The aging of the whole population as well as of the labor force in most of the industrialized countries–although the level and speed of the aging process differs–to a high degree, is, besides declining fertility, the result of increases in life expectancy in older adult life. This positive development is expected (at least in principle) to continue in the future. Not only because of financing of social security, but also from a more general point of view, the reallocation of lifetime between work and retirement is already on the political agenda in many countries, including Germany. A comprehensive, integrated, and long-term oriented approach is needed which involves economic policy, especially labor-market policy, education policy, and fiscal and social policies. Early political decisions seem appropriate in order to give employees and employers a signal on changing conditions and allow them to adapt, for example, to new legal rules. This will become one of the major political topics at the beginning of the new millenium in countries with aging populations.

NOTES

1. For details, see Bundesministerium des Innern (n.d.) and Enquete-Commission (1998), Chapter 1.

2. In Schmähl, George, and Oswald (1996), the different options in Germany for exit from the labor force for older workers are described. See also Boersch-Supan and Schnabel (1998) for figures on the declining labor force participation of older male employees and the incentive effect of the social security scheme. A detailed discussion on labor-force participation and social security is given in Schmähl (1989).

3. Costs of these strategies were mostly externalized, resulting above all in higher contribution rates in unemployment and pension insurance, resulting on the other hand in demands for reducing contribution rates because of their effect on labor costs.

4. This is in line with the recent experience that increases in life expectancy mainly are the result of reductions in mortality in higher adult age groups (the curve of survivors increasingly approaches a rectangular shape); Vaupel and Lundstrom (1996).

5. This is not determined by demographic conditions alone but especially also by labor-market conditions in combination with institutional rules regarding coverage, for example.

6. Basic information on the concept and structure of statutory pension insurance in Germany (covering old age, disability, and survivors) is given in Schmähl (1993).

7. Philipson and Becker (1998) argue that such schemes reduce mortality, especially via additional possibilities to invest in health human capital, and thereby increasing costs of social security. There is a vast literature on determinants of mortality, a complex and often confusing field which "requires a multidisciplinary approach" (Murray, Lincoln, & Chen, 1992). One of the factors discussed is income; see, e.g., Duleep (1986). The effects of income-dependent life expectancy and possible distributional effects of measures implemented will not be discussed here.

8. I do not discuss the underlying assumptions for these statements, which are politically relevant, whether well founded by facts or not. Some aspects concerning competitiveness are discussed in Schmähl, 1995; for incentive effects in case of financing by taxes versus insurance contributions, see Schmähl, 1998b.

9. Different options are outlined in Schmähl, 1987 and 1989, or Chand and Jaeger, 1996, and Daykin and Lewis, 1999.

10. Quantitative effects as well as possible problems resulting from the development are discussed in Schmähl, 1997 and 1998a.

11. Lee and Skinner, 1999, generally suggest ". . . that the appropriate policy response . . . should depend on the causes of the problem" (p. 135). "One possible policy response to increased longevity and improved health functioning is to increase the retirement age. . . ." (p. 136).

12. There exist different views on the future development of the mortality-morbidity nexus; see for example, Lee and Skinner, 1999. In the German discussion, mostly positive assumptions concerning further improvement in health conditions and disability-free additional years in retirement for future cohorts are supported by cross-sectional empirical data. But there is a lack of longitudinal data giving cohort-specific information as a base for calculating unbiased effects.

13. The U.S. government has decided to increase "normal" retirement age for the full pension up to the year 2022.

14. However, not only labor supply is decisive, but also labor demand. This is much more difficult to predict. For Germany, this topic is discussed extensively in Enquete Kommission, 1998.

REFERENCES

Aaron, H. J., Bosworth, B.P., & Burtless, G. (1989). *Can America afford to grow old? Paying for Social Security.* Washington, DC: Brookings Institute.

Aaron, H.J., & Reischauer, R.D. (1998). *Countdown to reform–The great Social Security debate.* New York: The Century Foundation Press.

Boersch-Supan, A., & Schnabel, R. (1998). Social security and declining labor force participation in Germany. *American Economic Review, 88*, 173-178.

Bovenberg, A.L., & van der Linden. (1997). Can we afford to grow old? Centraal Planbureau, Research Memoranda No. 134, The Hague.

Bundesministerium des Innern (n.d.). Modellrechnungen zur Bevoelkerungsentwicklung in der Bundesrepublik Deutschland bis zum Jahr 2040, Bonn.

Chand, S.K., & Jaeger, A. (1996). Aging populations and public pension schemes. International Monetary Fund, Occasional Paper 147, Washington, DC.

Daykin, C., & Lewis, D. (1999). A crisis of longer life: Reforming pension systems. Institute of Actuaries and Faculty of Actuaries, Dublin.

Disney, R. (1996). Can we afford to grow older? A perspective on the economics of aging. Cambridge, MA: MIT Press.

Duleep, H.O. (1986). Measuring the effect of income on adult mortality using longitudinal administrative record data. *Journal of Human Resources, 21*, 238-251.

Enquete-Kommission "Demographischer Wandel." (1998). Zweiter Zwischenbericht, Bundestags-Drucksache 13/11460, Bonn.

Lee, R., & Skinner, J. (1999). Will aging baby boomers bust the federal budget? *Journal of Economic Perspective, 13*, 117-140.

Murray, C., Lincoln, J.L., & Chen, C. (1992). Understanding morbidity change. *Population Development Review, 18*, 481-503.

OECD. (1999). *Labor Force Statistics, 1977-1997.* Paris: Author.

Philipson, T.J., & Becker, G.S. (1998). Old-age longevity and mortality-contingent claims. *Journal of Political Economy, 106*, 552-573.

Schmähl, W. (1987). Social policies for reducing demographically induced costs in social security. *European Journal of Population, 3*, 439-457.

Schmähl, W. (1989). Labor force participation and social pension systems. In P. Johnson, C. Conrad, and D. Thomson (Eds.), *Workers versus pensioners: Intergenerational justice in an ageing world* (pp. 137-161). Manchester and New York: Manchester University Press.

Schmähl, W. (1990). Demographic change and social security. *Journal of Population Economics, 3*, 159-177.

Schmähl, W. (1993). The "1992" reform of public pension in Germany: Main elements and some effects. In *Journal of European Social Policy, 3*, 39-51.

Schmähl, W. (1995). Social security and competitiveness. In International Social

Security Association (Ed.), *Social security tomorrow: Permanence and change* (pp. 19-28).

Schmähl, W. (1997). Alterssicherung–Quo vadis? In *Jahrbuecher fuer National oekonomie und Statistik, 216*, 413-435.

Schmähl, W. (1998a). Insights from social security reform abroad. In R. D. Arnold, M.J. Graetz, and A.H. Munnell (Eds.), *Framing the Social Security debate: Values, politics, and economics* (pp. 248-271 and 280-286). Washington, DC: Brookings Institution Press.

Schmähl, W. (1998b). Financing social security in Germany: Proposals for changing its structure and some possible effects. In S.W. Black (Ed.), *Globalization, technological change, and labor markets* (pp. 179-207). Boston, Dordrecht, London: Kluwer.

Schmähl, W., R. George, & C. Oswald. (1996). Gradual retirement in Germany. In L. Delsen and G. Reday-Mulvey (Eds.), *Gradual retirement in the OECD countries* (pp. 69-93). Aldershot, Brookfield, United Kingdom: Dartmouth.

Vaupel, J.W., & H. Lundstrom. (1996). The future of mortality at older ages in developed countries. In W. Lutz (Ed.), *The future population of the world–What can we assume today?* (Revised 1996 edition) (pp. 278-296). Laxenburg: International Institute for Applied Systems Analysis.

"The Full Monty" and Life-Long Learning in the 21st Century

James H. Schulz, PhD

Brandeis University
Waltham, Massachusetts

KEYWORDS. Older workers, technological change, unemployment, job turnover, retraining

In the former Soviet Union, there was no unemployment. Everyone of age had a job. Unfortunately, the Soviet central planning process that ran the country was not able to get large numbers of workers into the jobs most needed by the economy. The result was superb job security and a huge waste of economic manpower.

In the United States and other industrialized countries, the opposite occurs–high job insecurity but much less manpower waste. Unemployment insurance was introduced in the West to deal with the loss of jobs, and pensions were introduced to deal with unemployability related to age. But

James H. Schulz is Associate Dean, Professor of Economics, and Kirstein Professor of Aging Policy at the Heller Graduate School, Brandeis University. He is author of *The Economics of Aging* (7th ed., Auburn House, in press) and co-editor of *Social Security in the 21st Century* (Oxford University Press, 1998). This article is a revised and expanded version of an address by James Schulz to the Association for Gerontology in Higher Education on the occasion of his receiving the 1998 Clark Tibbitts Award. It is dedicated to Juanita Kreps, the late Harold Sheppard, and the late Clark Tibbitts.

James Schulz can be contacted care of the Heller Graduate School, Brandeis University, Waltham, MA 02454-9110 (E-mail: schulz@brandeis.edu).

[Haworth co-indexing entry note]: "'The Full Monty' and Life-Long Learning in the 21st Century." Schulz, James H. Co-published simultaneously in *Journal of Aging & Social Policy* (The Haworth Press, Inc.) Vol. 11, No. 2/3, 2000, pp. 71-82; and: *Advancing Aging Policy as the 21st Century Begins* (ed: Francis G. Caro, Robert Morris, and Jill R. Norton) The Haworth Press, Inc., 2000, pp. 71-82. Single or multiple copies of this article are available for a fee from The Haworth Document Delivery Service [1-800-342-9678, 9:00 a.m. - 5:00 p.m. (EST). E-mail address: getinfo@haworthpressinc.com].

one major problem that has not been addressed well is job insecurity arising from jobs and skills that become obsolete. In America, "obsolete workers" whose unemployment benefits have run out and are too young for retirement are pretty much on their own in dealing with the problems that arise.

Life-long learning of skills that can be used in the "new jobs" is one of those ideas that many people talk about but few people take seriously. It is very much like early retirement where, again, everyone voices concern about its harmful aspects and then goes on to ignore them.

The lack of serious commitment to life-long training opportunities and the great enthusiasm about early retirement are intimately related. Unions, government, and business think it is cheaper to terminate workers at early ages than to retrain them for the new jobs being constantly created.

To understand why life-long training is not popular, one must first understand the basic cause of job termination in contemporary society. Karl Marx said that the key to understanding unemployment was the capitalists' need for a "reserve army" of unemployed workers to keep wages low and profits high. Marx's view is insightful, especially in light of Chairman Alan Greenspan's tenure at the Federal Reserve Board of Governors. In the 1990s, Greenspan has frequently pointed out a need to head off a yet-to-appear inflation that he has warned is lurking just around the next economic corner. Thus, in recent years, the Fed has deliberately dampened job growth, fearing an excessive reduction in unemployment.

EFFICIENT MARKETS, CONSTANT OBSOLESCENCE

But there is an even more fundamental basis for understanding job terminations, one not quite so sinister. To explain that basic source of unemployment, it is instructive to look at the economic history of cotton textiles in the United States.

In 1793, an American, Eli Whitney, invented the cotton gin–a machine to separate cotton fibers from the seed. Before this invention, it took one person about one day to remove the seeds from one pound of cotton. With Eli Whitney's cotton gin, a worker could produce not one but 50 pounds of cotton each day–a spectacular rise in productivity. As a consequence, American cotton became much more competitive on world markets, and most human jobs "separating cotton" disappeared.

The bulk of the early American cotton production went to England to be turned into textiles. England was the first country to industrialize, and cotton played a major role in the process. Textile factories were built all across the English countryside. But the jobs were not to last. Eventually, England lost out to the new technology and competitiveness of the mills in the North of the United States. But these mills then eventually lost out in the 20th century to newer mills with better equipment and cheaper labor in the American South. And the workers displaced, especially the older workers, found it difficult to adjust. More recently, the entire United States has been losing textile jobs to mills in India, China, and various other developing countries.

Here, then, is the dilemma. Economic efficiency (i.e., the optimum allocation of economic resources to maximize production and consumer satisfaction) means that various jobs are constantly made obsolete. *Technological changes* typically result in a demand for workers with different skills and make jobs in various industries obsolete. *Shifting preferences* of consumers, as a result of new products and shifting relative product prices, also make some jobs obsolete. Moreover, changes in the competitive advantage of different individuals, regions, or countries (what economists call *comparative advantage*) change labor demand in various regions and countries. Together these three sources of change (technology, consumer preference, and comparative advantage) mean no job is really secure. No worker can predict what will happen in his or her lifetime. Nor can workers easily shield themselves and their families from the insecurities generated.

When factories and machines become obsolete, we discard them. But what do we do when humans become obsolete? The hit movie *The Full Monty* dramatizes the social, economic, and psychological impacts that can occur when jobs are lost. The movie focuses on the desperation of a group of men who cannot find work after the local steel mill in a small British town shuts down. The magnitude of shame and desperation, after fruitless job searches, pushes these men ultimately into becoming strip-teasers and executing "the full Monty"–that is, revealing "it all." An inability to find a job in their community causes them to overcome the strong inhibitions and embarrassment of being seen naked in public (especially by friends and neighbors). The movie graphically shows the powerful forces that caused these men to turn, first, to crime and then to stripping (where the market indicated there was ample money to be made in this unusual profession).

GOVERNMENT AND THE MARKETS

Governments, however, can provide some protection from the insecurity that arises from market forces. And history shows that both workers and business owners subjected to strong competitive threats are quick to turn to the government for help.

However, government in such a situation is confronted with a dilemma. It generally wants to help its citizens deal with the problems arising from impersonal markets. But if government protection simply ignores the realities of changing technology, shifting preferences, and competition–the nation's general level of production and living standards will ultimately suffer. A task confronting all countries is to provide reasonable economic security to populations without sacrificing too much economic growth. The most appropriate policies to do this are not obvious. Hence the debate continues all over the world with regard to trade and tariff policies and social protection programs.

James Fallows has put it well in his classic article about the impact of foreign competition on the American steel industry in the 1970s and early 1980s. Foreign competition caused plant closings in the Chicago/Great Lakes region, an area that was to become known as the "rust belt." Here, at the time, was the densest concentration of steel mills in the world. But these steel companies "disdaining to undercut each other's prices . . . practically invited an attack by foreign producers who would compete on price" (Fallows, 1985). Fallows graphically describes the tragic devastation that fell upon many workers and their communities.

While Fallows understands and appreciates the key contribution to economic growth that market forces make, he uses the example of big steel to warn us of the tremendous power for change (good and bad) unleashed by these markets:

> Capitalism is one of the world's more disruptive forces. It can call [through its market forces] every social arrangement into question, *make cities and skills and ranks merely temporary.* To buy into it is to make a commitment to permanent revolution that few political creeds can match. [emphasis added]

If we think, as Fallows suggests, of market economies as revolutionary forces, it suggests the magnitude of the challenge we face in talking about providing workers with life-long training opportunities. If that need arises in part from the constantly changing nature of the workplace and jobs, then revolutionary markets create a learning and training challenge of huge proportions.

MEASURING JOB LOSS

Economists have measured the magnitude of the recent "job revolution." In one of the best studies to date, the Center for Economic Studies has estimated job destruction and creation rates for the manufacturing sector of the United States economy (Davis, Haltiwanger, & Schuh, 1996). The findings indicate that rates of change for the 16-year period spanning 1973 through 1988 were incredibly high. On average, about one in five manufacturing jobs was either destroyed or created *each and every year*–with about one in 10 jobs disappearing and slightly fewer being created.

A fourth source of joblessness, recession, is illustrated by Federal Reserve policy. The Fed's efforts to stop the double-digit inflation of the early 1980s through tightened monetary policy resulted in a recession of major proportions. The U.S. Bureau of Labor Statistics (BLS) estimates that about 11 million workers were displaced over the 1981-1985 period (Horvath, 1987). More recent BLS data (Farber, 1997) indicate that despite the sustained economic expansion over recent years, job-loss rates over 1993 to 1995 were the highest since 1981 (when data first began to be collected). "About 15 percent of U.S. workers were displaced from a job at some time during this three year period [1993-1995]" (Kletzer, 1998). Using data from the "Health and Retirement Study," Couch (1996) focuses on older workers ages 51 to 61, documenting the problems of finding new jobs and the lost-earnings levels when new jobs are found.

As the history of textile manufacturing indicates, however, this phenomenon of job loss and gain is not new–it has been present since the beginnings of the Industrial Revolution. For example, Kevin O'Rourke and Jeffrey Williamson (1999) point out that the late 19th century was also characterized by what we now call "globalization." During those earlier years, there was mass international migration of workers, rising integration of capital markets, and a rising income gap between the rich and poor in Europe–quite similar to the situation today.

Thus, in a fundamental way, job displacement and unemployment are a necessary evil in America's economic growth success story.

A ROLE FOR GOVERNMENT

Workers over the decades, then, have become well aware of the continuing threats to their jobs and have often taken action to try to prevent the losses. Some of the "solutions" offered have been:

- Reducing hours in the full-time work week to share work with the unemployed,
- Opposition to free trade agreements (such as NAFTA),
- Union negotiations or strikes to promote job security,
- Early retirement schemes to encourage older employees to leave the labor force, and
- Worker opposition, sometimes violent, to the introduction of new technology.

All these actions and others have been tried, but in the long run to little avail–at least in competitive market economies. They were up against a strong consensus among consumers, business, and government–particularly given what Charles Lindblom has called "the privileged position of business" (Lindblom, 1977). The majority accept the need for change (which produces job loss), seeing these changes as the key to the success of markets in promoting economic growth and higher standards of living. Higher living standards are seen to depend on the constant "revolutionary" change that Fallows talks about as characterizing market economies.

Despite the great economic gains to be reaped from allowing markets to operate relatively freely, there is a role for government and public policy in making the situation of workers and their families better. There are important issues to be debated and options to be chosen. A national commitment to life-long training opportunities is one of them.

Why do we only give lip service to the idea of learning throughout one's lifetime? First, there is a widespread belief that the wonders of science have created a situation where there is no longer enough work for everyone. Technological innovation and modern production methods–such as mass production, new energy sources, complex machines, and robotics–are seen as creating a surplus of workers. Many people argue that nations should recognize the reality of "surplus labor" and spread the available work around, creating a shorter work week and promoting earlier retirement–so that people can enjoy the leisure and wealth of what Galbraith (1958) called "the affluent society." Given the seemingly unlimited desire of people (even rich ones) for more products and services, economists argue that this view is erroneous; scarce resources (including labor) will never be sufficient to keep up with growing consumer demands. But the idea of labor surplus as a result of technological revolutions remains strong among almost everyone else. In such a world of labor surplus, there would seem to be no need for workers to retrain, especially as they get older–given that there is no shortage of workers.

Even if a need develops, the view is often that older workers are not as likely to be suitable for the new jobs, because everybody knows "you can't teach an old dog new tricks" (Yankelovich, Skelly, and White, 1985).[1] And even if you could, most employers view older workers as less productive and more costly than alternative sources of labor–such as the nation's youth, middle-aged women returning to the workforce, and workers in developing countries. Thus, it is not surprising that age discrimination is still rampant in the United States, that various types of retirement incentives became the biggest employee benefit of the 20th century, that workers are skeptical about the value of learning and training in the later years, and that, therefore, little remedial training takes place.

However, the attitudes and actions just summarized related to older worker characteristics and productivity are not so much the result of research and fact as they are of prejudice and ignorance. To the extent that there has been research, it in large part contradicts the prevailing views of employers. As Sterns and McDaniel (1994) point out, "an extensive body of research indicates that age and job performance are by no means highly correlated. If performance does anything with age, it improves slightly, but the relationship is very weak. This is true regardless of whether performance is measured by supervisory ratings or though other more objective productivity measurements."

Technological change and robotics have not made most human employment unnecessary. Older workers can learn and can be as productive as young workers, bringing to the job insights and wisdom that come with years of experience. Policies to retire workers at increasingly earlier ages do not come cheaply–as the current concerns about financing public and private pensions demonstrate.

WHAT TO DO

Despite the ignorance and prejudice that prevails, there are things that can be done that will improve the situation and that also have a reasonable chance for implementation. Caro and Morris (1992-93) list six major reasons why the United States should "make retraining older workers an increasingly important national need":

- Population aging with fewer young workers,
- Accelerating technological change,
- Greater corporate layoffs of middle-aged and older workers,
- Improved health in the later years of life,
- Inadequate income in old age for some, and
- Rising collective demands of older persons for improved employment access.

As Robert Reich has pointed out, "a national economic strategy that puts people first is not an outgrowth of ideology or a continuation of campaign sloganeering. It is a hard-nosed response to economic reality. U.S. competitive strategy must be based on the American workforce because the people are the only resource that remains in any meaningful sense 'American'" (Reich, 1994).

Back to Basics

In support of Reich's viewpoint that we need to invest in workers is a survey of more than half a million employees. When asked to rank the most important factors that influence their decision to stay or move from a job, respondents placed "opportunity to learn new skills" at the top (AARP, undated). In contrast, the amount of money received from a job ranked much lower.

First, there is the continual need to encourage a focus on the basics of education. Individuals need to improve or learn skills that can be used as they move from one job to another and that will help minimize the disruption of job changes. Writing, entrepreneurship, computer operation, financial planning, and good health practices are all important skills that are often inadequate. Rosabeth Moss Kanter (1994) agrees that companies need flexibility in hiring and firing policies. But she argues that, at the same time, there should be an explicit commitment to actions in the workplace that focuses *not* on promoting "narrow skills to fill today's slots" but on providing abundant learning opportunities to promote *increased* competence with age.

Today, there is great concern about the quality of education being received by our children and about whether they will be able to function in the jobs of the future. There is a major effort under way to improve the teaching of basic skills and to meet the needs of high-skill industries. There is general agreement that America should not emphasize industries dominated by low-skill jobs–industries increasingly serviced by low-paid workers in developing countries.

What we need to do is add to this effort of better educating our youth for entry-level jobs. We also need to commit nationally to updating those skills over time. Workers educated before 1980, for example, will not have had in their youth any formal schooling in computer literacy. Now they need to acquire that literacy and improve any other basic skills that are weak, so that they are better able to compete for specific jobs when they become unemployed. "Back to Basics" courses should be available to people of all ages. Research to date clearly shows that people have the ability to learn at any age and that education is a major asset in seeking reemployment at "living wages." Both employers and workers need to change their attitudes about learning the basics. Learning the basics should not stop at any age, and public/private policies should encourage it.

Promote More Competition in Education

The second major thing we can do is to use the competitive mechanisms that "cause" unemployment to also help solve the reemployment problem. As industrialized countries go, the United States is at the extreme end of the unemployment/training continuum–placing most of the costs, insecurity, and responsibility for finding a new job on the worker him or herself. At the other end are countries like Sweden, Japan, and Germany, where successive governments have taken a leadership role in establishing model education and training programs as workers move in and out of different jobs. France,

Australia, and Singapore promote employer-financed training through a payroll tax; in France, for example, employers must certify that at least 1.4% of payroll goes to training, or they must pay the difference into a publicly administered fund (Moore, 1996).

In contrast, in the United States, workers lose their jobs, often with little or no warning, and typically find themselves forced to fend for themselves. The federal government gives huge tax subsidies to encourage people to save for retirement and to retire early, but it gives very little in the way of incentives for people to seek out the education and training they need to work longer. Likewise, we pour billions of dollars into educational institutions but minimize competition (especially at the K-12 level) by our system of taxing people for education and then dividing up the money among a selected list of public institutions. People with modest or low incomes are thus given little opportunity to seek out what they think are the most suitable educational situations.

Caro and Morris (1992-93) state that "community colleges appear to be the country's most important resource for older worker retraining." (See also Bass & Barth, 1992.) Community colleges cost less to attend, are locally situated, have experience working with employers and responding to their needs, and have pioneered courses for older persons–both workers and retirees. Caro and Morris call for demonstration funds to encourage community colleges and other educational institutions to develop training programs.

More directed government money in this area is certainly needed. But there is also a need for more competition in education. As David Osborne (1999) observes, "it doesn't always take competition to spark innovation. But, particularly in the larger [school] districts, bureaucracy stifles all but the most capable and persistent reformers." The way to bring about that competition is to put more education money into the hands of the consumers and to treat education less like a government regulated, nationalized industry.

This raises the controversial topic of vouchers and educational choice. Today, that discussion is polarized into two opposing camps. However, a middle way needs to be found.

Clearly, society should encourage investment by individuals in education at all ages–when people are young, before workers lose their jobs, when they lose their jobs, and when homemakers want to return to the labor force. Government should institute a variety of tax incentives and grant programs that fund workers, not trainers. Let the educators and the trainers then compete for the workers' dollars.

An Example of a Successful Program: SCSEP

The Senior Community Service Employment Program (SCSEP) was legislated as part of Title V of the Older Americans Act (amended). Persons participating in the program must be age 55 or older, unemployed, and at an income level that is not more than 125% of the official poverty level. The program employs these people in a wide variety of part-time community services: health care, nutrition programs, home repair, weatherization and beautification, fire prevention, conservation, and restoration efforts.

While general administration of the program is by the U.S. Department of Labor, this department delegates the actual operation to a number of national sponsoring organizations and government agencies (such as the National Council on the Aging and the U.S. Forest Service). Rules allow monies available to be used for training; however, in fact, few are devoted to this activity. Most of the efforts go into creating community jobs for participants and matching participants with existing jobs that are unsubsidized by the program.

The SCSEP has been a popular program in the Congress, receiving significant increases in funding over the years. However, the number of older workers actually involved is still quite minimal (about 80,000 people in fiscal 1993). And it is estimated that less than one percent of those eligible for the program are able to participate, given current funding constraints.

The SCSEP program represents the beginnings of a comprehensive program for training and employing older workers. But it is far too limited and should be significantly expanded.

Attitudes Toward Retirement

One of the aging field's great pioneers, Clark Tibbitts, argued that society needs to rethink what individuals do with their lives in later life. He was a vocal advocate for expanded opportunities, both traditional work and non-traditional volunteer activities in the later years. He could not understand why society wanted to push older people into the proverbial "rocking chair"–even if it was a Boeing 747 headed for Hawaii. Clark Tibbitts saw later life as a time of learning and experimentation–a time for new roles, giving to one's community, and adapting to the job flexibility opened up by the income security provided by contemporary public and private pensions.

The distinction between work and leisure has blurred considerably in modern society. Yet the workplace, work rules, and employer attitudes have remained almost as rigid as ever. Not that there has been no progress. N. P. Eurich (1990) estimates ("guesses," she says) that around $60 billion was spent by businesses on training and retraining each year in the late 1980s, but another estimate says that two thirds of that training went to persons ages 25 to 45 (Carnevale, 1989). However, mandatory retirement has been abolished; increasing number of employers are hiring older people for part-time or part-year jobs, and millions of older people currently volunteer their time to help others.

A CONCLUDING THOUGHT

At the beginning of this article it was said that we in the United States only give lip-service to life-long training opportunities. That is not totally correct. There is no way any of us can go through life without constantly learning. Much of that learning directly relates to the ability to function in different jobs. The challenge is to heighten awareness of that fact, to harness our learning capacities to better meet the many challenges of life (such as the tragedy of unemployment), and to remember that learning comes in lots of different forms–with access never to be limited by age.

NOTE

1. For an alternative view of older persons as learners, see Bass and Barth (1992).

REFERENCES

AARP. (n.d.). *Preparing for an aging work force–A practical guide for employers.* Washington, DC: Author.

Bass, S., & Barth, M. (1992). *The next educational opportunity: Training for older adults.* Background paper series. New York: The Commonwealth Fund.

Carnevale, A.P. (1989). The learning enterprise. *Training Development Journal,* 27-35.

Caro, F.G., & Morris, R. (1992-93, Dec/Jan). Retraining older workers: An emerging economic need. *AACC Journal,* 22-26.

Couch, K.A. (1996). Late life job displacement. *The Gerontologist, 38,* 7-17.

Davis, S., Haltiwanger, J., & Schub, S. (1996). *Job creation and destruction.* Cambridge, MA: The MIT Press.

Eurich, N.P. (1990). *The learning industry: Education for adult workers.* Princeton, NJ: The Carnegie Foundation for the Advancement of Teaching.

Fallows, J. (1985, March). America's changing economic landscape. *The Atlantic Monthly,* 47-58.

Farber, H.S. (1997). The changing face of job loss in the United States, 1981-1995. *Brookings Papers on Economic Activity.*

Galbraith, J.K. (1958). *The affluent society.* Boston: Houghton Mifflin.

Horvath, F.W. (1987, June). The pulse of economic change: Displaced workers of 1981-1985. *Monthly Labor Review,* 3-12.

Kanter, R. M. (1994). U.S. competitiveness and the aging workforce: Toward organizational and institutional change. In J.A. Auerbach and J.C. Welsh (Eds.), *Aging and competition: Rebuilding the U.S. workforce.* Washington, DC: National Council on Aging.

Kletzer, L.G. (1998, Winter). Job displacement. *Journal of Economic Perspectives, 12,* 115-136.

Lindblom, C.E. (1977). *Politics and markets*. New York: Basic Books.

Moore, T.S. (1996). *The disposable work force*. New York: Aldine De Gruyter.

O'Rourke, K., & Williamson, J. (1999). *Globalization and history: The evolution of a 19th century Atlantic economy*. Cambridge, MA: MIT Press.

Osborne, D. (1999, October 4). Healthy competition: The benefit of charter schools. *The New Republic*, 31-33.

Reich, R.B. (1994). A global, technological economy. In J.A. Auerbach and J.C. Welsh (Eds.), *Aging and competition: Rebuilding the U.S. work force*. Washington, DC: National Council on the Aging.

Sterns, H.L., & McDaniel, M.A. (1994). Job performance and the older worker. In S.E. Rix (Ed.), *Older workers: How do they measure up?* Washington, DC: Public Policy Institute, AARP.

Yankelovich, Skelly and White, Inc. (1985). *Workers over 50: Old myths, new realities*. Washington, DC: AARP.

An Aging Workforce
in an Increasingly Global World

Michael C. Barth, PhD

ICF Consulting
Fairfax, Virginia

KEYWORDS. Employment, American labor force, mid-career workers, older workers, global markets

Two of the salient features of our millenial world are its aging population (at least in the industrialized nations) and the globalization of markets. People, goods and services, information, and capital move with great speed to the locations in which they contribute most to output. Most economists agree that the result of the newly internationalized allocation of resources is positive, but sometimes with undesirable distributional effects.

Mid-career and older workers are concerned both with the world in which they work and the world in which they will retire. Regarding the latter, economic and social conditions that increase national output are unambiguously good. That is, retirees' focus is on the ability of the social insurance system to provide income and health care in line with expectations. If a world of open borders for people, goods and services, information, and capital leads systematically to higher output–which I take as a given–then it is this world

---

Michael C. Barth is Executive Vice President, ICF Consulting, 9300 Lee Highway, Fairfax, VA 22031 (E-mail: mbarth@icfconsulting.com). He directed The Commonwealth Fund's Americans Over 55 at Work Program and has published widely on issues relating to older workers. Prior to joining ICF in 1980, he was Deputy Assistant Secretary for Income Policy, U.S. Department of Health and Human Services.

[Haworth co-indexing entry note]: "An Aging Workforce in an Increasingly Global World." Barth, Michael C. Co-published simultaneously in *Journal of Aging & Social Policy* (The Haworth Press, Inc.) Vol. 11, No. 2/3, 2000, pp. 83-88; and: *Advancing Aging Policy as the 21st Century Begins* (ed: Francis G. Caro, Robert Morris, and Jill R. Norton) The Haworth Press, Inc., 2000, pp. 83-88. Single or multiple copies of this article are available for a fee from The Haworth Document Delivery Service [1-800-342-9678, 9:00 a.m. - 5:00 p.m. (EST). E-mail address: getinfo@haworthpressinc.com].

of relatively open borders that is most likely to be able to meet, or disappoint least, the retirement needs of millions of American baby boomers. In addition, should a retiree in the United States wish to return to work, his or her ability to do so will depend on the state of economic conditions and his or her own skills relative to those needed in the job market. There is, therefore, reason for near-retirees and retirees to favor a politics that supports globalization, as well as employer behavior that gives older people a fair shake. Finally, the older person will need to ensure that he or she is ready for the job.

In this essay, I explore the relationship between the aging American labor force and an increasingly international world. I am interested in the requirements of this world for mid-career and older workers, and in the benefits of this world for the next life-course stop of these workers–retirement. First, I sketch the most relevant characteristics of the new global markets, searching out the implications for workers. Then, I review what we know about employers' views of older workers in order to see how these perceptions accord with the skill and attitude requirements of jobs. The concordance is imperfect, and leads to suggestions for actions and policies that might facilitate the adaptation of older workers to the global world. I conclude by noting the arguments for why older people should support globalization at the macro level and suggest specific policies and behaviors at the micro level.

WORKER REQUIREMENTS

A world of relatively open borders has the following relevant characteristics:

- *More competition.* Since many products can be produced almost anywhere, there are few protected markets (of any consequence).
- *Rapid change.* Since information and investments move with great speed, change is a constant. Where change is a constant, there is a premium on adaptability.
- *Emphasis on entrepreneurship.* Change yields openings for new ideas. If capital to finance the new ideas is available, entrepreneurs will move rapidly to create and capture new markets.
- *Internationalization of production.* The last 15 years or so have seen large and not-so-large businesses going abroad to reduce production costs and to be near customers. This tendency will accentuate labor skill differences among nations, at least in the short run. High-skill countries, like the United States, will become the producers of relatively more skill-intensive products. Products requiring lower-skill workers will be produced elsewhere.

- *Use of the latest technologies.* The free flow of information, combined with competition, ensures that, subject only to high capital costs, producers around the world will use the latest technologies.
- *More economic growth.* Holding constant the skills of the world's monetary and fiscal policymakers, the internationalized world should be more efficient and produce more, leading to real income growth. In the near term, income growth will be more evident in the economies with the most ideal combination of wise policies and open markets.

In this stylized world, what are the ideal characteristics of workers? In a world characterized by competition, entrepreneurship, and rapid change, the most important characteristics of workers would seem to be flexibility, adaptability, and the ability to use new technology.

EMPLOYER VIEWS OF OLDER WORKERS

During the last 15 years, there have been at least four nationally representative surveys of employers that asked their views of the strengths and weaknesses of older workers (AARP, 1985; AARP/DYG, 1989; Mirvis, 1993; SHRM/AARP, 1998). In these studies, older workers were defined as age 50 plus. In the aggregate, the managers interviewed rated older workers highly on the following:

- Experience
- Commitment to quality
- Low turnover
- Attendance/punctuality
- Judgement

Managers rated older workers as relatively weaker (or less desirable) on the following:

- Flexibility
- Acceptance of new technology
- Ability to learn new skills
- Physical ability to perform strenuous jobs
- Contribution to health care costs

Often it is thought that the lists of positives and negatives offset each other, leaving employers somewhat neutral in their views of older workers. This was decidedly not the finding of the one study (of which I am aware) that was able to explore with managers the relative importance of their pro/con views of older workers (AARP, 1995; this study was performed for AARP by ICF Consulting and directed by the author of this paper). While this study's data comes from 12 case studies of companies (and one state government), I believe the results are compelling because, when asked questions that were quite similar to those that appeared on the nationally representative surveys, the respondents provided answers that are remarkably similar to those found in the national surveys.

We asked *which traits were most highly desired for the future* by managers. The answer: flexibility, adaptability to change, and a capacity and willingness to exercise independent judgement. These are, unfortunately, among the traits attributed to older workers by managers as weakness.

It is instructive to compare the traits managers value more–flexibility, adaptability to change, and acceptance of technology–with those they value less–experience, punctuality, low turnover. Surely, having workers who show up on time and who do not quit frequently must be important. Managers agree, but add that they must respond very quickly to changes in competitive conditions the world over. Not everything can be *most* important. Managers want employees who are best at what the manager perceives to be his or her greatest challenge. A review of the characteristics of the global business world confirms that the managers' views are logically consistent.

Without attention to overcoming these negative perceptions, some older workers will face a bleak future.

PUBLIC AND PRIVATE POLICY

What can be done to align workers with the realities of the modern global workplace? Workers themselves, employers, and government all have roles to play. Workers can actively stay abreast of the latest workplace technologies and innovations and seek training and places on teams formed to develop and implement new methods for getting the work done. They can avoid behaviors that, anecdotally, are frequently mentioned by employers as indicators of older workers' technological inhibitions: not choosing direct deposit of paychecks and an inability to master the video cassette recorder. They can enroll in computer training courses, learn to "surf the Net," and, at work, discuss what they have learned.

Employers must provide mid-career and older workers with training opportunities. The AARP study cited above (AARP, 1995) found that a vicious circle exists that begins when employers tend to exclude mid-career and older workers from training, making them unable to perform new jobs, which, in turn, makes them appear unable to adapt. A conflict exists between the time needed for employers to achieve a target rate of return on training investments and the equity implications of excluding a group from training. This conflict cannot be wished away. Workers must do all that is in their power to make employers think that training *them* will be an investment worth its cost. The few studies of worker productivity that were able to compare workers of different ages suggest that older workers have much to offer at no added cost (see Hogarth & Barth, 1991; McNaught & Barth, 1992). Indeed, in both of the companies studied, older workers required *less* training time than originally planned and no more than normally provided to younger workers. Employers might also observe the enormous costs of recruitment as they contrast the far lower turnover rates of older workers compared with those of their younger colleagues.

Government can play a research and development role by supporting studies whose goal is to make available hard data and analysis on the questions for which there are strong opinions but relatively little analysis: How do older workers respond to new technology and to the pace of technological innovation? How do older workers assimilate job-related training? What are the impediments to adaptability in the workplace? Both data-based research and demonstration or experimental studies would be valuable in each of these areas. Significantly, government must enforce anti-discrimination policies and should examine carefully the allocation of training opportunities. Training can be critical to a worker's future. Not having training opportunities may be one of the most powerful, if subtle, ways that a worker can be disadvantaged.

Aging advocacy organizations and labor unions can complement government activities by playing a major role in educating employers and the public about the productivity of older workers.

CONCLUSION

How should mid-career and older American workers view the internationalized world? The answer depends upon their age, their skills, and their income and health care needs in retirement. If, as I asserted earlier, the internationalized world leads to greater economic growth in the United States, then people closer to retirement should view internationalization more favorably. The longer one wishes to work, and the more marginal one's skills, the more problematic this dynamic, global workplace will be.

American labor union and liberal political groups have, in general, tended to oppose globalization, as, for example, in their positions on the North American Free Trade Agreement and on immigration quotas for skilled workers. If my assertion that globalization will enhance U.S. economic growth is valid, retirees will certainly benefit from it. It is in the closing years of their work lives that older workers face a conflict. A sensible way to deal with the conflict would be for older workers, and their employers, to make the "cost" part disappear by taking the steps suggested here.

REFERENCES

American Association for Retired Persons. (1985). *Workers over 50: Old myths, new realities.* Washington, DC: American Association for Retired Persons.

American Association for Retired Persons/DYG. (1989). *Business and older workers: Current perspectives and new directions for the 1990s.* Washington, DC: Author.

American Association for Retired Persons. (1995). *Valuing older workers: A study of costs and productivity.* Washington, DC: Author.

Hogarth, T., & Barth, M. (1991). The costs and benefits of older workers: A case study of B&Q's use of older workers. *International Journal of Manpower, 12*(8),5-17.

McNaught, W., & Barth, M. (1992, Spring). Are older workers "good buys"?: A case study of Days Inns of America. *Sloan Management Review, 33,* 53-63.

Mirvis, P. (Ed.). (1993). *Building a competitive workforce: Investing in human capital for corporate success.* New York: John Wiley & Sons.

Society for Human Resources Management and AARP. (1998). SHRM/AARP Older Workers Survey.

LONG-TERM CARE

Continuing Care Retirement Communities and Efficiency in the Financing of Long-Term Care

John A. Nyman, PhD

University of Minnesota

KEYWORDS. Long-term care, continuing care retirement communities (CCRCs), Medicaid, annuities

Continuing Care Retirement Communities (CCRCs) are firms that sell housing and long-term care services to the elderly. In exchange for a large fixed payment (or "endowment") and a smaller monthly fee, CCRCs agree to provide housing, maintenance, some cleaning services, some food, and

---

John A. Nyman is an Economist and Professor in the Division of Health Services Research and Policy, School of Public Health, University of Minnesota. He has written extensively on nursing home and long-term care policy.

John A. Nyman can be contacted care of the Division of Health Services Research and Policy, School of Public Health, University of Minnesota, 420 Delaware Street, S.E., Box 729, Mayo, Minneapolis, MN (E-mail: ihsr@tc.umn.edu).

[Haworth co-indexing entry note]: "Continuing Care Retirement Communities and Efficiency in the Financing of Long-Term Care." Nyman, John A. Co-published simultaneously in *Journal of Aging & Social Policy* (The Haworth Press, Inc.) Vol. 11, No. 2/3, 2000, pp. 89-98; and: *Advancing Aging Policy as the 21st Century Begins* (ed: Francis G. Caro, Robert Morris, and Jill R. Norton) The Haworth Press, Inc., 2000, pp. 89-98. Single or multiple copies of this article are available for a fee from The Haworth Document Delivery Service [1-800-342-9678, 9:00 a.m. - 5:00 p.m. (EST). E-mail address: getinfo@haworthpressinc.com].

(often) long-term care services to elderly persons or couples for the rest of their lives. During the initial years, when the elderly residents are relatively healthy, the CCRC may operate at a surplus for that resident, or couple, but if and when the resident's health declines and he or she must be admitted to the nursing home wing of the CCRC, the CCRC may operate at a deficit for that person. The pooling of revenues from many residents and prudent actuarial management, however, allow the CCRC to remain solvent.

In recent years, the financing of long-term care for the elderly has become a major policy issue. Public financing through Medicaid has become increasingly burdensome, but private financing options–such as long-term care insurance–are often regarded as too expensive and, therefore, lack the volume necessary to relieve much pressure from Medicaid. A number of government programs have been suggested to either subsidize existing long-term care insurance, or provide government-sponsored insurance at subsidized prices. The problem with many of these programs is that they require additional government funds. Instead of introducing policies that increase government subsidies, an alternative approach may be to introduce policies that allow the elderly to use their existing resources more efficiently. The promotion of CCRCs is one such policy.

THE RISK TRANSFER ADVANTAGE OF CCRCS

CCRCs have a number of efficiency advantages over other ways of financing long-term care services. First, CCRCs allow the elderly person to make more efficient use of his or her financial resources by assuming the financial risk for housing, food, and care needs for the rest of that person's life. That is, few of us know when we are going to die. We may know that on average persons aged 65 are expected to live another, say, 15 years, but an individual aged 65 would be foolish to spend down his or her own resources at a rate such that, by the end of the 15 years, nothing was left. A prudent individual must always spend at a lower rate because of the possibility that he or she might live longer than expected.

If a person buys an annuity, he or she can make more efficient use of his or her resources because annuities allow one to transfer this risk of living longer to the annuity company. In exchange for a lump-sum payment, an annuity company will promise to pay a certain amount per month for the rest of one's life. The amount that the annuity company agrees to pay depends largely on the purchaser's life expectancy. If the annuitant, that is, the purchaser of the annuity, lives longer than expected, the annuity company loses money; if the annuitant dies earlier than expected, the annuity company does not have to pay as much as expected and ends up with a surplus. Because the annuity company sells annuities to a large number of people, it can rely on the law of large numbers to balance losses with surpluses, and make disbursements predictable. The purchasers of the annuity, however, make more efficient use of their resources because they have eliminated the need to keep some resources in reserve in case they live longer than expected. It is as if they have more resources to spend.

At least in theory, CCRCs represent annuities that pay off in kind. In exchange for a certain large endowment payment (and the smaller monthly fee), the CCRC agrees to provide room, board, and long-term care services as needed until the end of life. Again, it is as if the person who buys a CCRC contract has more resources because he or she has transferred to the CCRC some of the risk of having unexpected consumption expenditures. As a result, the individual can afford better accommodations and amenities with a CCRC contract than without.

In addition to the annuity, CCRCs also provide long-term care insurance. Like an annuity, insurance enables an individual to make more efficient use of his or her resources. This is because, in contrast to reserving (or saving) resources to pay for the eventuality of long-term care, the person buying insurance can take advantage of the relatively small probability of needing long-term care to buy insurance for a certain amount of long-term care expenditures at a fraction of that amount as the premium (de Meza, 1983; Nyman, 1999). For example, a person who wants $100,000 in long-term care coverage may only need to pay premiums of a total of $30,000 if financed by insurance because the probability of loss is 30%. If an individual wants to finance such an expenditure from his or her own resources, it would require reserving the entire $100,000 from the consumption stream. Financing the eventuality of long-term care through insurance means the person thus has more spendable resources and can afford to spend more on both long-term care and other consumption.

An individual who buys only long-term care insurance makes efficient use of some of his or her resources. In contrast, one who buys a CCRC contract makes efficient use of more resources because the CCRC provides long-term care insurance, plus an annuity that in theory can cover housing, food, maintenance, and some housekeeping needs as well. That is, because expected living expenses are included, the person with the CCRC annuity makes efficient use of more of his or her resources than someone who has merely bought long-term care insurance, and is therefore able to afford more.

HOUSING SERVICE DUPLICATION ADVANTAGE

The second way CCRCs make more efficient use of resources is that they enable an individual to avoid the need to pay for two sources of housing services at the same time. Many elderly enter nursing homes directly from their homes. They retain possession of their homes because, if they do recover from their nursing home stay, they want to be able to return home. While this is understandable, it is also expensive: The elderly person is occupying two sources of housing services–their house and a room at the nursing home–at the same time. Clearly, if the elderly person were to rent out their house during the time they were in the nursing home, there would be more resources available to purchase nursing home care or to purchase care with more amenities, but this is rarely done. More often than not, the house stands vacant while the elderly person relies solely on his or her nonhousing resources to pay for nursing home care. As a result, the cost of retaining a primary residence while in a nursing facility represents an "opportunity cost"–a cost incurred by not taking advantage of renting out the house–to the individual. To society, however, it represents a real cost because additional housing resources are needed to accommodate those who could have purchased housing services from the nursing home resident.

In contrast, people typically sell their houses before entering a CCRC. Once in a CCRC apartment, if the elderly person's health deteriorates to a sufficient extent, he or she is transferred to the nursing home wing of the CCRC. At that point, the apartment that this individual was occupying becomes available for someone else. To make this arrangement agreeable, there are typically provisions in CCRC contracts–provisions for accommodating very short nursing home stays, spouses, and the possibility that the person may be able to return to another apartment after a longer-term nursing home stay–that cover the exceptions. The upshot, however, is that the person who buys a CCRC contract does not occupy two housing sources simultaneously, and the contract can therefore afford to include more amenities in both the apartment and nursing home.

ANOTHER SOURCE OF EFFICIENCY

Another source of efficiency is the scale and other economies that are realized because the CCRC delivers home health services to those who are living on the CCRC site. If someone requires personal care services at home, this often requires a specific contract with a caregiver, who often must travel a substantial distance to perform these services. Moreover, the recipient may not require that all the services be performed at once, but be spread over a number of hours, during which the caregiver has some down time. In contrast, residents of CCRCs may receive care from a caregiver who is already at the CCRC, on an ad hoc basis. Delivery of services in this way is likely to be less costly than conventional delivery.

Because of the availability of personal and other services for persons living in a CCRC apartment, residents with declining health may also remain in apartments longer than they otherwise would have been able to do. This implies that CCRC residents may be able to avoid costly nursing facility care longer than others. Sloan, Shayne, and Conover (1995) found evidence that persons whose CCRC contracts were capitated for nursing home care had significantly lower nursing home use than those whose CCRC contracts incorporated nursing home care payments on a fee-for-service basis. This suggests that the capitated aspect of some CCRC contracts provides an incentive for the CCRC to keep persons out of expensive nursing facilities longer than they would under conventional circumstances. Indeed, Sloan, Shayne, and Whetten-Goldstein (1995) found that CCRC residents' functional, cognitive, and health status declined at a slower rate than did the status of elderly persons in other living arrangements. While these results may reflect selection, they may alternatively reflect efficiencies in outcomes that are due to the quality of the services delivered. It should be noted that, while keeping CCRC residents healthier and out of the CCRC's nursing facility longer are efficiencies from society's perspective, they may require additional CCRC costs because the residents live longer.

CCRCs AND MEDICAID

In theory, expected Medicaid expenditures would likely be reduced when an elderly person signs a CCRC contract. This is because with a CCRC contract, the purchaser has likely converted assets held as a private residence into assets held as claims against the CCRC. Because of this conversion, additional assets are available to pay for services that would otherwise be paid for by Medicaid.

In 1993, the Omnibus Budget Reconciliation Act (OBRA) mandated that states increase their efforts to recoup Medicaid funds spent on behalf of the beneficiary from the beneficiary's estates. For example, a typical scenario might be as follows. An unmarried person without dependents is admitted to a nursing home. At some point in her stay, the patient is deemed a permanent resident of the nursing home, and at that point, the assets represented by her primary residence are no longer excluded. With OBRA, states would be required to recover the Medicaid expenditures from the value of the home, either by placing a lien on the house or making a claim against the value of the house during probate after the Medicaid recipient dies. Sabatino and Wood (1996) surveyed state Medicaid programs regarding their estate recovery practices and found a great deal of unevenness in the level with which states were complying with OBRA '93. Moreover, a major and growing segment of the legal profession now practices "elder law," which is often devoted to finding legal loopholes that would permit the client to retain, transfer, or bequeath the home, while still qualifying for Medicaid.

The amount of additional assets at stake could be substantial. In 1992, the median net worth for those aged 75 and over was $87,000 (Kennickell, Starr-McCluer, & King, 1994). Of all those in this age group, about 70% held at least some of their assets in a primary residence. The median value of these primary residence holdings was $55,900. If the net worth for all those aged 75 and over households is representative of the net worth of those aged 75 and over who own homes, this would suggest that the median elderly person of this age needed to spend down only about 36% of total wealth to qualify for Medicaid.

In contrast, the typical person or couple who enters a CCRC has already sold their home, so there are no housing assets–about 64% of the typical elderly person's net worth–to exclude. As a result, the person in a CCRC must therefore exhaust about three times the amount of assets–from both housing and nonhousing sources–to qualify for Medicaid, compared with the person who enters a nursing home directly from his or her home. This suggests that fewer persons would qualify for Medicaid if they were in CCRCs than if they were living in their homes. It further suggests that Medicaid expenditures would be reduced to the extent that the elderly bought CCRC contracts.

From a CCRC's perspective, when the value of a person's house is excluded in determining Medicaid eligibility, Medicaid has imposed a disincentive–namely, the value of the person's house in the form of a transfer or bequest–to the purchase of a CCRC contract. In order to make a level playing field, it would be necessary to give persons entering a CCRC a subsidy of commensurate value to the Medicaid subsidy embodied in any de facto house exemption.

Wiener, Illston, and Hanley (1994) reviewed the options on financing long-term care for the elderly and proposed to increase government involvement by subsidizing long-term care purchases. Their proposals were motivated by the logic that (1) private long-term care financing is difficult because all the options are so expensive, and (2) Medicaid provision requires impoverishment and, thus, stigmatizes the recipient. The political problem with increased subsidization of long-term care is that if government were to pay for private long-term care purchases outside of Medicaid, it would simply be acting to preserve an estate. Therefore, the beneficiaries of such programs would be largely the heirs of those estates, not the frail elderly.

CCRCs may represent a policy solution to the long-term care financing problem. First, CCRCs make the most of the elderly person's own resources, enabling the elderly to purchase more and better housing, food, and long-term care services than they would otherwise have been able to afford. In other words, the package of services–including long-term care insurance–provided in a CCRC arrangement may be less expensive (in terms of present consumption or other assets forgone) to the individual than the same package would be if these services were financed directly through income, savings, or the liquidations of other assets. Second, CCRCs reveal that Medicaid–far from being a bare-bones program that requires impoverishment–is actually quite generous, often allowing persons the unnecessary luxury of occupying two sources of housing services simultaneously. Understandably, many elderly may be so attached to their homes that they do not want to part with them. The choice to retain ownership of one's home and risk going on Medicaid rather than use one's resources more efficiently by buying a CCRC contract, however, is the individual's. A public subsidy (in the form of allowing persons to bequeath their home to their heirs rather than spending its value on their care) should not be used to make this inefficient choice more attractive.

WHY ARE THERE SO FEW CCRCs?

Currently, there are many fewer CCRCs than nursing homes. A person's attachment to his or her own home and the Medicaid housing exclusion may explain some of the sparseness on the demand side. On the supply side, CCRCs encounter problems that have tended to make them risky businesses (Conover & Sloan, 1995/96; U.S. Senate, 1983).

First, although they function like insurance companies by assuming risk, CCRCs have far fewer customers on which to base their expected cost projections. As a result, they cannot depend on the law of large numbers to reliably predict their expenditures. This has meant that CCRC business failures have been relatively common in the past. Moreover, for those CCRCs that have recognized this problem and attempted to accumulate sufficient reserves by pricing conservatively, their sometimes large surpluses have made them targets of tax litigation by county assessors who want to take away their tax-exempt status. This, too, has made their expenses difficult to predict.

Second, CCRCs may encounter adverse selection, but often lack the actuarial sophistication or underwriting capability to adjust for it. Adverse selection may manifest itself in CCRCs in two ways: (1) by admitting people who are healthier–those who are likely to outlive their expected lifetimes–than the general population, and (2) by admitting fewer persons with terminal diseases than are in the general population. (Persons with terminal diseases would be reluctant to forgo the initial endowment payment for an expected short-term stay in a CCRC, yet they would be included in the health distribution of the general population.) If persons who are healthier than average are admitted, but cost estimates and revenue needs are based on general population life expectancy and nursing home use projections, the CCRC may encounter financial difficulties.

Admitting residents on a first-come, first-served basis appears to be a common practice. Empirical evidence suggests that CCRCs may experience some selection bias. Sloan, Shayne, and Whetten-Goldstein (1995) surveyed CCRC residents in 1992 and found that persons admitted to CCRCs had fewer functional impairments and chronic health conditions at entry than non-CCRC elderly, but interestingly that CCRC admissions were more likely to have cancer than non-CCRC elderly. It is not clear why this increased prevalence of cancer exists.

Third, CCRCs in theory allow elderly to remain independent as long as possible by providing incrementally more care services to them as their health status declines, but allowing them to remain in their apartments as long as possible. Accordingly, CCRC patients are likely to exhibit slower declines. As mentioned above, Sloan, Shayne and Whetten-Goldstein (1995) found that CCRC residents had acquired fewer activities-of-daily-living needs, were better cognitively, and had acquired fewer chronic health conditions than non-CCRC elderly. This suggests the impact of CCRCs on resident health is to extend their longevity, but this may also increase the CCRC's financial risk.

PRACTICAL LIMITATIONS

The foregoing analysis suggests that CCRCs have a number of advantages over other forms of long-term care financing that make them a desirable public policy option. There are a number of limitations, however, that may make them less desirable in practice than they are in theory.

First, CCRCs are not all alike. Some do not provide the extensive "life care" feature that commits them to provide care services to residents for the rest of their lives, including nursing home care. Some may be owned and run by unscrupulous persons who raise the monthly fee exorbitantly over time, reduce services and amenities, or even default on their contracts. Others may be able to cream-skim the most lucrative cases, increasing their profitability, but diluting the public policy attractiveness of these contracts.

Second, CCRCs are not pure annuities: the required monthly payments means that not all of the end-of-life risk is transferred to the CCRC. These monthly payments may be large enough to cover the entire apartment living costs for a relatively healthy individual without tapping into the value of the amortized endowment revenue stream. In such a case, there is little annuity value to the endowment payment, which would then merely represent a one-time-only long-term care insurance premium. Moreover, although a large portion of these payments is likely to be financed by Social Security and other pension benefits, there might also be some small portion of the monthly payment that must be paid for out of pocket.

Third, Medicaid eligibility requirements under OBRA 1993 may be enforced less aggressively in some states, or the states may have lax estate-recovery programs, which increases the subsidy that the housing exclusion represents. This may decrease the appeal of CCRCs vis à vis Medicaid financing because if long-term care is financed through Medicaid, the person's house may become part of his or her bequest.

Fourth, Medicaid covers home health care in many states, and home health care would also allow the less dependent Medicaid beneficiary to avoid using two sources of housing services at the same time. Other options, such as reverse mortgages and assisted living, may incorporate some of the same efficiencies. The availability of such options would decrease the uniqueness and attractiveness of CCRCs.

Despite these practical considerations, CCRCs represent a potentially attractive policy solution to the long-term care financing problem, and one that clearly deserves a closer look. The central challenge is to develop policies that will promote the creation of CCRCs with all the features that should allow the elderly to finance their own long-term care affordably and efficiently.

POLICY RECOMMENDATIONS

Government policy toward CCRCs could proceed in a number of directions. One might be to adopt policies aimed at better leveling the playing field by making certain that private housing assets are used to finance an individual's long-term care first, before resorting to Medicaid. Any ability to avoid the spending of one's own housing assets creates a disincentive *not* to join a CCRC.

Alternatively, government might become involved in solving the practical issues associated with CCRCs. For example, government could encourage the merger of CCRCs to increase the size of the resource pool. Or, it could sponsor programs to educate CCRCs on actuarial and underwriting techniques so as to better price their contracts. Or, it could provide a reinsurance program so that CCRCs would have access to greater risk-sharing.

Or, government might sponsor studies of the various options available to make both (1) better use of hitherto unused housing assets of the elderly and (2) more efficient use of existing resources by converting them to annuities. These options would include policies directed at CCRCs, but they might also include assisted living, reverse mortgages, long-term care insurance, and other options.

Efficiency in the delivery of long-term care services has long been a policy goal. A large number of studies has been conducted to determine the setting where long-term care could be delivered least expensively (Weissert, 1988). Efficiency in the financing of these services is at least as important, but has received much less policy attention. With the possibility of being able to stem, and potentially reverse, the growth of Medicaid expenditures, financing arrangements that shift the burden to the patient and extend the patient's own resources are clearly attractive. Because continuing care retirement communities may be unique in being able to achieve both of these goals simultaneously, they deserve another look.

REFERENCES

Conover, C. J., & Sloan, F.A. (1995/96 Winter). Bankruptcy risk and state regulation of continuing care retirement communities. *Inquiry, 32*(4), 444-456.

DeMeza, D. (1983, March). Health insurance and the demand for medical care. *Journal of Health Economics, 2*(1), 47-54.

Kennickell, A. B., Starr-McCluer, M., & King, T.W. (1994, October) Changes in family finance from 1989 to 1992: Evidence from the Survey of Consumer Finances. *Federal Reserve Bulletin, 80*(10), 861-882.

Nyman, J. A. (1999, April). The value of health insurance: The access motive. *Journal of Health Economics, 18*(2), 141-152.

Sloan, F. A., Shayne, M. W., & Whetten-Goldstein, K. (1995). Health and functional status of the elderly in continuing care retirement communities versus other settings. Unpublished manuscript.

U.S. Senate, Special Committee on Aging. (1983). *Life care communities: Promises and problems.* 98th Congress, 1st Session, May 25, Washington, DC: USGPO.

Weissert, W. G. The national channeling demonstration: What we knew, know now, and still need to know. *Health Services Research, 23*(2), 175-187.

A Special Consumer Cooperative Association Nursing Home

Masato Oka, MSc

KEYWORDS Nursing home, consumer cooperative association, workers, collective, welfare-mix, Japan

A unique welfare facility for the elderly in Japan, named the "Rapport Fujisawa," is the subject of this article. It is a mixed facility consisting of a special nursing home and an in-home care support center for the elderly. It was established in May 1994 by an innovative Japanese consumer cooperative association called the Seikatsu Club Seikyo Kanagawa (henceforth, SCSK). "Seikatsu" means life, "Seikyo" means consumer cooperative, and "Kanagawa" is a prefecture close to Tokyo.

HISTORY AND BACKGROUND

SCSK started its retail business in 1971. It has had no stores, but has been distributing safe food and eco-friendly daily goods directly to the members through a small neighborhood group of 5 to 10 members called the "HAN," which coordinates advanced booking of joint purchases and distributes the goods (Yokota, 1991, p. 23f). As of FY 1996, the membership was 47,150 households belonging to 8,080 HAN members. There were 11 regional

---

Masato Oka is Professor at the Economic Research Institute, Yokohama City University, Yokohama, Japan. He is co-author of *Regulating Employment and Welfare: Company and National Policies of Labor Force Participation at the End of Worklife in Industrial Countries* and *A Welfare Vision of Independence and Choice.* He was Guest Editor of a 1996 issue of the *Journal of Aging & Social Policy* (Vol. 8, No. 2/3) on public policy and the old-age revolution in Japan.

[Haworth co-indexing entry note]: "A Special Consumer Cooperative Association Nursing Home." Oka, Masato. Co-published simultaneously in *Journal of Aging & Social Policy* (The Haworth Press, Inc.) Vol. 11, No. 2/3, 2000, pp. 99-106; and: *Advancing Aging Policy as the 21st Century Begins* (ed: Francis G. Caro, Robert Morris, and Jill R. Norton) The Haworth Press, Inc., 2000, pp. 99-106. Single or multiple copies of this article are available for a fee from The Haworth Document Delivery Service [1-800-342-9678, 9:00 a.m. - 5:00 p.m. (EST). E-mail address: getinfo@haworthpressinc.com].

branches with a total of 252 employees. The annual total sales was 18.36 billion yen (U.S. $153 million, if $1 is 120 yen) and the total amount of invested capital by members was 3.86 billion yen (U.S. $32.2 million). The average monthly sales per household (31,972 yen or U.S. $266) and the amount of invested capital per household (81,731 yen or U.S. $681) were the highest of all Japanese cooperatives (Oka, 197, pp. 20-21).

The members of the SCSK have been mostly young and middle-aged educated housewives. Under the slump-inflation after the first oil crisis of 1973, they had become quite sensitive to social, economic, and political issues. They had gradually enlarged their activities from the joint purchase of daily goods to concern for ecological, peace, social welfare, and political reform issues (SCSK, 1991, p. 153f).

The activities of SCSK related to attempting to cope with the aging society started in the early 1980s. The leaders explained the reasons as follows. First, the members recognized the fact that they themselves would be living in the aged society of the early 21st century, in which one fourth of the total population would be 65 and older. Second, they thought that the spirit of mutual help and the community network of the cooperative association should be the basis of constructing a life-support system for the elderly (Kimura, 1996, p. 20).

The first action was organizing a "workers' collective" (or a workers' cooperative association) named "Group Tasukeai" (Group Mutual Help) in 1985 in Yokohama. It is a kind of nonprofit organization in which all members take part in investment and management, and work in the home help and care services. This new work system has been developing rapidly. As of 1996, there were 34 sister workers' collectives in Kanagawa Prefecture, with the membership of 3,000 supplying more than 200,000 thousand service hours mainly for the household of older persons (Kanagawa Workers' Collective Rengo Kai, 1996, p. 11f; Do, 1997).

The second action was founding a kind of mutual insurance system for SCSK members in 1986. The members pay a small monthly premium, and at the time of illness or injury home health services are provided by other members. The fund pays a reasonable remuneration for their work. This system has also been effective in developing a spirit of mutual help among the members (SCSK, 1991, pp. 228-229).

The third action was the establishment of a day service facility named "Seikatsu Rehabilitation Club Asoh" in 1987 in Kawasaki City, the second largest municipality in Kanagawa Prefecture. It was the first experiment for the consumer cooperatives in Japan. Later, three more facilities were opened in order to be centers for community welfare. The Kawasaki municipal government has contracted out day services to the facilities mentioned (Kimura, 1996, p. 21).

CONSTRUCTION OF THE RAPPORT FUJISAWA

In 1991, commemorating the 20th anniversary of SCSK, its annual General Meeting proposed a plan to construct a welfare facility for the elderly named the "Rapport Fujisawa." Fujisawa is the name of a municipality with a population of 360,000, located 30 miles southwest of Tokyo. The reason Fujisawa was chosen might be its convenience and comfortable location as well as SCSK's close relationship with the progressive Fujisawa municipal government, which recognized SCSK as a good partner for improving social services in the aging society.

A theoretical key concept of this partnership was called "community optimum." The concept was developed through the following historical process. Since the late 1950s, the Japanese national government had tried to build a welfare state based on the British concept of "national minimum." It aimed at providing a minimum standard of decent life for all. However, it was far from the ideal goal because of financial limitation and bureaucratic constraints. Since the middle of the 1960s, progressive local governments of large municipalities had tried to improve the system with additional social services based on the concept of "civil minimum," setting more ambitious goals toward a welfare community. It was successful for a while in meeting people's growing needs; however, after the first oil crisis of 1973, those local governments had faced financial difficulties due to the rapid increase of service costs and decreased revenue. At the same time, people became greatly concerned about not only more efficient social services but also more participation in the decision-making process. Replying to this need, the new concept of "community optimum" was developed. The basic idea was that people's needs should be met with optimum conditions in the community in which they lived through the collaboration of relevant actors, including the national and local governments, nonprofit organizations, private enterprises, and individuals and families (Ishige, 1986; SCSK Education Bureau, 1997, p. 47).

For the Rapport Fujisawa project, SCSK needed to raise funds of more than 200 million yen (U.S. $1.7 million) out of the total estimated construction costs of 1,500 million yen (U.S. $12.5 million). The leaders proposed that SCSK meet one half of 200 million yen with its accumulated surplus, and another half with donations from members. The initial response of members was not so positive. They preferred using their fund to improve their own lives rather than using it for unknown older people. The top leaders repeatedly explained the aims of the new facility, as follows: First, the facility should be a community welfare center backed by the active participation of members. Second, it would be run by joint work among the members of workers' collectives and professional workers. Third, it should disclose all information to relevant people and organizations, and jointly share the challenges of making a community welfare model. Through hot and long debate, the leadership of SCSK was finally successful in persuading members to recognize the importance of the project for their own future. Moreover, in this campaign process, members' interests in workers' collectives providing home help services had steadily increased and new associations were successively established (Kimura, 1996, pp. 21-22; interviews with Ms. Y. Kimura and Mr. K. Yokota).

There was one more big issue to be solved. The Kanagawa Prefecture Government initially insisted that the basic fund for establishing a social welfare juridical person for the Rapport Fujisawa should not be contributed by many and unspecified persons because there was no such precedent. After negotiation of several months, the government finally accepted the new method of fund raising through collective efforts of small benefactors. The target of funding was completed in three years' time with the donation from 70,000 people (ibid).

The final total cost of the project was 1,485 million yen (U.S. $12.4 million) including the cost of land (24.5%), the construction cost of the facility (73.6%), and the cost of the fund to run the facility (1.9%). In regard to the cost sharing, SCSK and its group contributed a total of 218 million yen (U.S. $1.8 million) or 14.8% of the total cost. The remaining cost was covered by subsidies from the national and local governments (56.2%), a low-interest public loan (28.7%), and a donation from a charity fund (0.3%) (ibid).

THE FACILITY AND FUNCTIONS

The facility of the Rapport Fujisawa is a three-storied building with a gross floor area of 2,644 square meters in the site area of 3,310 square meters. There are a total of 30 rooms with 70 beds, including 10 single rooms, 10 double rooms, and 10 quartet rooms. The fixed capacity is 50 beds for the residents and 20 beds for the short-stay service (IkiIki Fukushkai, 1996). In regard to the floor planning, a common living space for each three residential rooms was designed in order to provide a homey atmosphere for residents. The corridor leads to the common space and then to the residential rooms. The government initially questioned this design, thinking it might produce a dangerous dead angle for caregivers. However, the original design survived with a slight modification. The common living space proved its effectiveness for producing a friendly group life among residents and caregivers (Kimura, 1996, p. 23).

The first function of the Rapport Fujisawa is a special nursing home for the elderly. Thirty residents with heavy senile dementia live on the third floor, and 20 residents without dementia live on the second floor. As of 1996, the average age of residents was 82, and the oldest resident was a 98-year-old woman. Most of the residents are frail, with complications (ibid, p. 24).

The second function is an in-home care support center to serve a population of 60,000 elderly people. The Fujisawa Municipal Government has been contracting out the following services: (1) in-home care support service provided by two experts; (2) day service, available for 25 elderly a day, Monday through Friday–the service users pay 500 yen (U.S. $4.20) for a lunch; (3) bathing service, available for bedridden elderly, free of charge–the local government gives a subsidy of 15,000 yen (U.S. $125) per case; (4) home-visit nursing care service, with service users paying 500 to 1,500 yen (U.S. $4.20 to $12.50) according to their income level; (5) emergency telephone call service–24-hour service for 730 elderly as of FY 1995; (6) meals-on-wheels service–a total of 5,300 meals were served in FY 1995 and a workers' collective has been engaged to provide the cooking service; (7) short-stay service–20 beds are available at 8,000 yen (U.S. $66.70) a night, of which 5,700 yen (U.S. $47.50) is subsidized; (8) home-help service–the number of service users in 1995 was 96, with an average age of 78.3 years (ibid, p. 23; and interview with Ms. Y. Kimura).

STAFF AND QUALITY OF SERVICE

As of 1996, the number of paid staff of the Rapport Fujisawa was 43, including 22 caregiving staff called "partners." In addition, cooking, laundry, and care-assistant services were provided by two workers' collectives with a total of 61 members. Volunteers, called "citizen partners," and one companion dog were collaborating with the staff just mentioned (ibid, p. 24).

The guidelines for care in the Rapport Fujisawa can be summarized as follows. First, an independent life style for each elderly person should be guaranteed as much as possible. Second, the remaining physical and mental capabilities of the elderly should be fully utilized. Third, the right of self-choice and the human dignity of the elderly should be fully respected (Rapport Fujisawa, 1996, pp. 4-5). The wording itself may be almost the same as that of advanced facilities in the world. However, it seems surely unique, as the services are being provided not only by professional workers but also by ordinary housewives belonging to the workers' collectives. The Kanagawa Prefecture Government initially was suspicious of the capability of workers' collectives to provide cooking and care services, and recommended that only professional workers be hired.

SCSK strongly insisted on the importance of ordinary people's active participation in the social services of the aging society. As a result, cooking and laundry services were contracted out to the workers' collectives. As for the care service, members of workers' collectives were individually employed as part-time workers. The head of the Rapport Fujisawa said that there was no serious problem as far as the relations between these "amateur" workers and the professional care staff (Kimura, 1996, p. 23, and interview).

Thirty members of the Workers' Collective Hana-momen (flower cotton) are quite sensitive regarding the serving of meals in the manner most suitable to each client. Another 31 members of the Workers' Collective Miyui (fruition) are engaging in laundry and care-assistant services to clients with the pride of housewives serving members of their families. Since they are living in the neighborhood area of the Rapport Fujisawa, these workers' collective members have lots of enjoyable local information for the elderly. Moreover, the community network of these housewives is useful when it comes to inviting local people to annual events at the facility, for example, an art exhibition. These "human-touch" services must be precious and priceless. It seems that the collective workers' devoted services greatly enrich the quality of services of the Rapport Fujisawa.

CONCLUDING REMARKS

The case of Rapport Fujisawa seems to suggest the possibility of a new mutual support system among citizens based on the ideal of cooperation. As Rapport Fujisawa is only five years old in 1999, it is too early to give a full evaluation of its activities and effects. However, at least it might be possible to say that it is an important experiment toward a goal of a new welfare-mix system based upon collaboration among nonprofit organizations and public bodies. The theoretical concept of "community optimum" seems to present a useful framework for the partnership.

What is the potential for replication of Rapport Fujisawa elsewhere in Japan and in other societies? Since its opening, many leaders of relevant organizations have been visiting it to learn about the experience and the reality. That shows the impact of the project; however, there has been no news that such a facility has been founded elsewhere in Japan. That suggests that it would not be easy to fulfill the necessary conditions for success.

The first condition would be the fund-raising capability. As mentioned earlier, the initial founding costs were funded by the accumulated surplus of SCSK and donations from 70,000 group members. It might be very difficult for ordinary consumer cooperative associations.

The second condition would be the human resources. The members of SCSK are mostly middle-aged intelligent housewives who are politically progressive and seeking opportunities for active participation in the life of their communities. They join the workers' collectives and enjoy their work of serving the elderly. However, they are still in the minority in the present

Japanese society, though it seems that this social consciousness of citizens has gradually been developing, especially in the urban areas.

The third condition would be a good relationship with the public bodies. The Kanagawa Prefecture Government and the Fujisawa Municipal Government gave full support to Rapport Fujisawa through subsidies and contracting out of various services. The main reason might be that the governors of both local governments were the prominent progressive leaders, insisting on the values of participatory democracy and decentralization of authority. They shared these values with the leaders of SCSK. However, again, this type of political leadership still is in the minority in the present Japanese political world. Therefore, the model would not be easily replicated elsewhere in Japan under the current situation. However, if the necessary conditions were satisfied with further development of the cooperative association, together with further progress of participatory democracy through positive political reform, there would be higher potential for replication of the model in the future.

REFERENCES

IkiIki Fukushkai (social welfare juridical person "Active Welfare Association"), (Ed.) (1996). *Rapport Fujisawa: Shisetsu Gaiyo.* (Introductory leaflet on the facility of the Rapport Fujisawa). (In Japanese).

Ishige, E. (1986). Tenkanki no shakafukushi gyousei to jichigata fukushi (The administration of social welfare and the participatory welfare system in the transitional period). *Bulletin of Iida Women's College.* Iida, Nagano. (In Japanese).

Kanagawa Workers' Collective Rengokai (Kanagawa Workers' Collective Union), (Ed.) (1996). *1995 nendo jigyou hokokusho* (Annual Report, FY 1995). Yokohama: Author. (In Japanese).

Kanagawa Workers' Collective Union. (1997). *New working system in the twenty-one century, Workers' Collective.* Yokohama: Author. (information pamphlet in English).

Kimura, Y. (1996, July). Nana man nin no shinrai: Rapport Fujisawa (Trust of 70,000 people: The Rapport Fujisawa). *JA Keiei Jitsumu* (Japan Agricultural Cooperative Association's Magazine on Management Practice), 19-24. (In Japanese).

Oka, M. (1997). Seikatsu Kyodo Kumiai (Consumers' cooperative association). In T. Ohuchi (Ed.), *Chiiki no fukusi sabisu kyokyu ni kakawaru hieiri minkan dantai no rodoryoku jukyu ni kansaru kenkyu* (A research report on the labor force of nonprofit organizations supplying social services in the local community), 13-24. Tokyo: Koyo Sokushin Jigyodan. (In Japanese).

Rapport Fujisawa (Ed.) (1996). *Chiiki ni kurasu, chiiki wo tsukuru; Rapport Fujisawa 2 shunen* (Living in a community, making a community: 2 years' anniversary of the Rapport Fujisawa). Fujisawa: Author. (In Japanese).

SCSK (Ed.) (1991). *IkiIki alternative: Seikatsu Club Kanagawa 20 nen no ayumi* (Twenty years' history of SCSK). Yokohama: Author. (In Japanese).
SCSK Group, Education Bureau (Ed.) (1997). *Vision no kyokasho* (Text book of vision/history). Tokyo: Author. (In Japanese).
Yokota, K. (1991). *I among others*. Tokyo: Seikatsu Club. (In English).

INTERVIEWS

Mr. Katsumi Yokota (the top leader of SCSK Group). May 1997 and April 1999.
Ms. Yoko Kimura (the head of Rapport Fujisawa). November 1997.

The Chronic Care Paradox

Robert L. Kane, MD

University of Minnesota School of Public Health
Minneapolis, MN

KEYWORDS. Chronic care, primary care, clinical pathways, decision-making

American medicine faces a paradox. As we enter the dawn of the 21st century, we continue to practice medicine in the style of the nineteenth. Albeit armed with access to major technological advances, we still seem to treat each encounter as a unique event, rather than components of a continuing process of care.

Although demographic and epidemiological studies clearly show that we are firmly in the era of chronic disease, we persist in acting as though we are still treating primarily acute illnesses. Over two thirds of the current health care dollar goes to treating chronic illness; for older persons, the proportion rises to almost 95% (Hoffman, Rice, & Sung, 1996). In the face of such evidence, it behooves contemporary medical practice to change its approach. We need to adopt a focus more appropriate to chronic disease.

A focus on chronic disease implies a number of changes in emphasis and

---

Robert L. Kane holds the Minnesota Chair in Long-term Care and Aging at the University of Minnesota School of Public Health, where he directs the Center on Aging and the Clinical Outcomes Research Center.

Dr. Kane can be contacted in care of the University of Minnesota School of Public Health, D351 Mayo (Box 197), 420 Delaware Street SE, Minneapolis, MN 55455 (E-mail: kanex001@tc.umn.edu).

This work was supported in part by a Geriatric Leadership Academic Award (#5K07-AG00622) from the National Institute on Aging.

[Haworth co-indexing entry note]: "The Chronic Care Paradox." Kane, Robert L. Co-published simultaneously in *Journal of Aging & Social Policy* (The Haworth Press, Inc.) Vol. 11, No. 2/3, 2000, pp. 107-114; and: *Advancing Aging Policy as the 21st Century Begins* (ed: Francis G. Caro, Robert Morris, and Jill R. Norton) The Haworth Press, Inc., 2000, pp. 107-114. Single or multiple copies of this article are available for a fee from The Haworth Document Delivery Service [1-800-342-9678, 9:00 a.m. - 5:00 p.m. (EST). E-mail address: getinfo@haworthpressinc.com].

107

thinking. New definitions are needed for such familiar concepts as prevention. Medical management changes, especially the goals for care. The role of patients changes dramatically. Time assumes a different meaning. Professional roles may change. Expectations about the benefits of care are altered.

While primary prevention is directed at the reduction of risk factors that can ultimately lower the likelihood of developing diseases, under the banner of chronic care, the preventive emphasis changes to respond to the WHO definition of the relationship between impairment and disability (WHO, 1980). Effective prevention will reduce the transition from disease to disability. Much of the success of medical care is measured less in terms of impressive saves, but rather in addressing chronic problems early in order to prevent the exacerbations that could lead to expensive care. Special emphasis is placed on avoiding iatrogenic complications.

In effect, more attention is placed on disease management, but the methods to achieve this end may vary. In the arena of chronic disease, reliance on clinical pathways and guidelines may be frustrating, because many patients have multiple chronic problems. Consensus about management for any one may be complicated by the other comorbidities. Instead of prescribing specific evaluative and therapeutic activities, it may prove more effective to require a structured information system. Specifically, a clinical glidepath approach may prove useful in managing chronic problems. Under this approach, one or two clinical parameters are identified for each condition. These are selected from a candidate list on the basis of the clinician's beliefs about which ones will best reflect the clinical status of that patient. For example, if a patient had congestive heart failure, one might want to monitor the extent of edema or the intensity of shortness of breath. The choice of sign or symptom would depend on how the disease manifested in a given patient. In many instances, the patients themselves may be able to provide the data directly, thus involving them more actively in their own care. These parameters are then tracked on a regular basis and compared to an expected clinical course. The expected course can be generated statistically from large data bases (when available), or it can be based on clinical judgment. Any statistically significant deviation triggers an alarm that alerts the clinician to the possibility of an incipient problem and invites early attention and a careful reappraisal of the clinical situation.

Figure 1 shows an example of a clinical glidepath. In this instance, the expectation is that the symptoms will improve over time. In the first several observations, the observed result is as good or better than expected. (The expected range is shown as a pair of dotted lines.) The last observation is outside the confidence limits. That level of deviation should trigger an alarm system to warn the clinician of a potentially serious course change. Figure 2 shows another example, akin to a recovery after a hospitalization; here the

FIGURE 1. An Example of a Clinical Glidepath Where the Expected Course Calls for Improvement

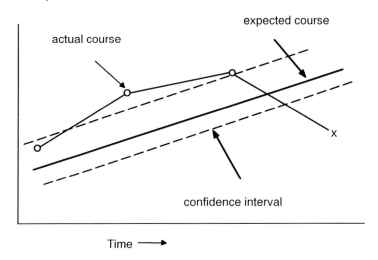

expected course calls for initial improvement and then a steady state. Here too, the early observations are within the confidence limits, but the last observation is outside them.

This technique suggests a special need for information systems that can track the status of designated clinical parameters for each chronic condition. Frequently collected data can be plotted against prognoses to identify when the patient's clinical course is deviating from the expected one.

Chronic illness implies a different role for patients, one that emphasizes more shared responsibility. Patients should play a greater role in clinical decision-making, having more say in what is done, but concomitantly accepting more responsibility for the outcomes. Patients must be more vitally involved in their own care for chronic problems. They are the ones most in touch with events on a day-to-day basis.

In order to make better decisions, patients need better information about the risks and benefits of alternative treatments. They need to establish more effective communication with their physicians. The clinical glidepath system described above provides a possible vehicle for such productive patient involvement. Many of the clinical parameters needed to monitor changes in disease status are symptoms. Patients could be productively used to systematically monitor these (as well as some signs such as blood pressure and blood sugar), recording them or transmitting them to computerized clinical records. Patients could actually be notified when the patterns indicate a potential problem and use this notification as a prompt to contact their physicians.

FIGURE 2. An Example of a Clinical Glidepath Where the Expected Course Calls for Initial Improvement Followed by a Steady State

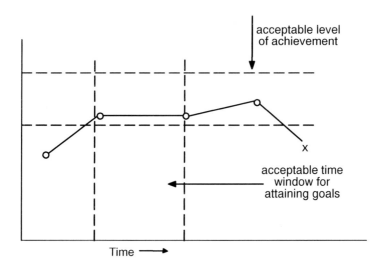

New developments in inexpensive programmable handheld computers and voice recognition systems suggest a means of facilitating clinical monitoring. The ability to structure a simple data base that patients (or their families) could enter regularly and transmit to a central location by modem offers a host of new opportunities for more closely tracking chronic problems. Likewise, home care workers could be supervised and instructed at a distance using this technology. Simple algorithms could drive data collection and even indicate the urgency of responses needed to changes in patients' status. Instructions could be updated over the telephonic connections.

The very notion of chronic disease implies a different role for time. Care is better measured in terms of episodes rather than events. Individual encounters do not define a clinical episode. Patients do not appear on the clinical radar screen only when they present for treatment. Rather, their status is more continually monitored.

Likewise, the timeframe for determining efficiency is shifted. A basic concept to be applied revolves around investment. In essence, greater attention to early problems (even at a greater initial cost) is justified if there is good evidence that such early interventions can prevent expensive exacerbations. Hence, more effort is devoted to comprehensive evaluations and active monitoring.

The basis for allocating clinicians' effort is also changed. Instead of relying on fixed allocations of time per encounter, the proportion of effort is determined by the nature of the patient's prior course. Patients who remain on their glidepath are likely to need only minimal attention, leaving the time saved to be devoted to those who are drifting off the prognosed pathways.

Chronic disease care invites a reconsideration of how professionals are used. There is a great opportunity to employ downward delegation at several levels. Nurse practitioners can provide a substantial component of primary care, especially in regard to overseeing the routine monitoring of disease status and following protocols for early intervention. At the same time, many nursing tasks can be delegated to nonprofessionals, making assistive services more affordable and available in locations such as assisted living facilities. Developments in electronic communication make it feasible to oversee the performance of such staff at a distance and to provide timely feedback as circumstances change.

New thinking is needed about who is best suited to provide primary care for patients with chronic disease. Despite the current enthusiasm for primary care providers, for the subset of persons with unstable or complicated conditions primary care may be best provided by specialists who can better manage these conditions. However, some of these specialists may not be comfortable managing patients as opposed to organ systems. In those cases, teams of specialists and nurse practitioners may represent the best approach.

A concomitant of chronic disease is long-term care. While only a fraction of chronic disease patients will require long-term care at any single point in time, the care for that subset is important. Good medical care is especially germane to this group. Effective coordination requires shared goals. Historically, long-term care has pursued a more compensatory course, developing means to address clients' lost functional ability, whereas clinical care has emphasized therapeutic goals, which pursue benefit. In fact, these two components are complementary and should both be directed toward therapeutic care. In the case of long-term care, positive therapeutic outcomes may be measured in terms of slowing the rate of decline. The achieved functional outcomes should be as good as or better than what is reasonably expected (Kane, 1995). Expectations can be derived statistically from large data sets or can be based on clinical judgments.

Making the transition from an acute care paradigm to one directed at chronic care will not be easy. Several steps are needed beyond simply articulating the challenge. New technologies, especially information technologies, need to be harnessed to support the transition. Commercially available patient tracking systems will expedite adoption. More projects that demonstrate the effectiveness of these new approaches will make them increasingly attractive. New graduates need to be trained to think in new paradigms, but extant practitioners will need special assistance in making the transition. While there will undoubtedly be some resistance, there is growing appreciation that the current system is not working.

Bringing about these changes will not be easy, because it involves changing basic assumptions and practice styles. The best motivation to change is a belief that the change is worth the effort, namely that the resultant savings or improved care will justify the disruption of routines. It would seem most feasible to look to organized practice situations to initiate the changes. Much of the current thrust to change practice has come under the aegis of continuous quality improvement, but this approach tends to be project focused. More tangible mechanisms, like the clinical glidepaths, are needed, at least to complement these efforts. One way to change practice may be to identify new practitioners, or to take advantage of emerging trends. For example, the growth in nurse practitioners as chronic care providers might introduce a new set of players more receptive to the chronic care model.

Before practitioners will embrace behavioral change, they must be shown that these changes improve care, and ideally save money. Carefully conceived demonstration projects are needed, primarily in the form of randomized clinical trials, to establish the effectiveness of new approaches.

Initially, there was reason to hope that managed care might prove the needed catalyst to facilitate the transition to chronic care. In theory, managed care should be well positioned to recoup the investment in making the changes through subsequently lowered costs of care that result from more effective care. Unfortunately, the potential of managed care organizations to serve as the locus for change has not been borne out. Despite the theoretical potential for managed care to benefit from the savings that better chronic care could produce, it has opted to emphasize short-term gains over longer-term investments (Kane, 1998). In the world of Medicare, managed care has done better by relying on favorable selection, being paid average costs and recruiting healthier than average clients (Brown & Hill, 1994). Such a strategy is diametrically opposite to one that addresses chronic care.

It thus seems unlikely that society can rely on market forces to bring about this transition. External pressures and inducements (including the results of studies that demonstrate the value) will be needed, at least to the point where the appreciated benefits confer a market advantage on those adopting the new precepts.

Medicare has a vital stake in facilitating the shift to a chronic disease model. It appears to have placed great faith in a managed care strategy, which was primarily pursued (perhaps mistakenly) as a cost containment device. Alternatively, Medicare could encourage better attention to chronic care more directly by rewarding such care under its fee-for-service reimbursement programs, but it appears that these programs are being phased out as quickly as possible in favor of various forms of prospective payment. Medicare has not been successful in finding ways to reward specific provider behaviors. The efforts with the Resource-Based Relative Value System (RBRVS) physician payment scheme have worked only modestly. Some form of special reward or acknowledgement for providers who employ an adequate intensity of chronic care techniques might be possible, but there is no precedent for such a step.

Two different strategies are thus open to Medicare to use payment incentives to improve chronic care. The first strategy addresses managed care. Under the current system, there is a strong disincentive for managed care organizations to become skillful at chronic disease management. They are currently much better off enticing a relatively healthy clientele. Were they to establish a chronic disease competence and attract a following of sick, disabled persons, they would be paid at a rate less than the actuarial costs of this group. The Health Care Financing Administration (HCFA) has announced its plans to change the managed care capitation calculation. It will rely on administrative data based on past Medicare billings. It recognizes that such an approach will likely underestimate the costs of caring for complex chronic care cases, but has postponed recommendations on the needed risk adjuster. The best candidate for such an adjuster lies in the realm of functional measures (e.g., ADLs and IADLs), but such data would have to be collected directly; they are not available from administrative records. HCFA seems loath to mandate direct data collection, either because it is too complicated or because it does not trust the providers to report the data accurately. However, there is already ample precedent for using provider-generated data to calculate Medicare payment rates (e.g., using the Minimum Data Set [MDS] as a basis for nursing home prospective payment or the Outcome and Assessment Information Set [OASIS] for home health care).

The second strategy is more difficult, that is, paying providers directly for better chronic care; but it might be worth some experimentation. One approach would simply pay providers more for managing more complicated cases. This approach would presumably reimburse for the extra time involved. It would be hard to monitor the actual increase in time and effort, especially if that effort were reflected in intensity rather than just time.

An alternative would be to pay some form of bonus for managing chronic conditions well. Such a program would require methods for both identifying patients with complex chronic needs and assessing the results of more effective care. The easiest way to measure the results would be in terms of preventing subsequent utilization of expensive care like hospitals and emergency rooms. Indexes of preventable hospitalizations have been proposed and used in evaluation studies (Billings, Anderson, & Newman, 1996; Bindman et al., 1995), but they have never been used as the basis for direct reward systems. An immediate problem is the limitations of small numbers; most clinicians will have only modest numbers of chronically ill patients, too few on which to calculate a stable rate that could be used as the basis of payment. Before such a scheme could be implemented, it seems appropriate to test the feasibility of one or more approaches.

Chronic care thus faces yet another paradox. While we can argue the need to recast the approach to care to accommodate the different needs of chronic care, it seems unproductive to advocate for major infrastructure changes in the care system until the payment system provides at least some support for such a revolution. It is hard enough to get medical providers to change their behavior; it seems Sisyphean to ask them to swim against the payment tide.

REFERENCES

Billings, J., Anderson, G. M., & Newman, L. S. (1996). Recent findings on preventable hospitalizations. *Health Affairs, 15*(3), 239-249.

Bindman, A. B., Grumbach, K., Osmond, D., Komaromy, M., Vranizan, K., Lurie, N., Billings, J., & Stewart, A. (1995). Preventable hospitalizations and access to health care. *Journal of the American Medical Association, 274*(4), 305-311.

Brown, R., & Hill, J. (1994). The effects of Medicare risk HMOs on Medicare costs and service utilization. In H. Luft (Ed.), *HMOs and the elderly* (pp. 13-49). Ann Arbor, MI: Health Administration Press.

Hoffman, C., Rice, D., & Sung, H.-Y. (1996). Persons with chronic conditions: Their prevalence and costs. *Journal of the American Medical Association, 276*(18), 1473-1479.

Kane, R. L. (1995). Improving the quality of long-term care. *Journal of the American Medical Association, 273*(17), 1376-1380.

Kane, R. L. (1998). Managed care as a vehicle for delivering more effective chronic care for older persons. *Journal of the American Geriatrics Society, 46*, 1034-1039.

WHO. (1980). *International Classification of Impairments, Disabilities, and Handicaps: A Manual of Classification Relating to the Consequences of Disease*. Geneva: World Health Organization.

Who Will Care for Mother *Tomorrow*?

Andy Van Kleunen, MA
Mary Ann Wilner, PhD

Paraprofessional Healthcare Institute
Bronx, New York

KEYWORDS Paraprofessional long-term care workers, home health aides, certified nursing assistants, frontline workers, direct care workers

Within the ongoing discussion of how to save Medicare and Social Security, there is an alarming silence about the looming crisis in long-term care. Few policymakers and politicians are hearing the question foremost in the mind of a family member of someone who needs long-term care: "Who will take care of Mother *tomorrow*?"

Anyone experienced in the long-term care system knows well the fear remote to the uninitiated, that the home care aide or nursing assistant will not arrive on time–or at all–to wash, assist, or feed Mother. Will she be someone Mother knows? Will she be kind and gentle? Competent and respectful? Will she be rushed, or have time to talk and listen?

Healthcare paraprofessionals–as Genevieve Gipson, the director of the National Network of Career Nurse Assistants, has so keenly observed–are "the point where the system touches the client." In the end, the *quality of the*

Andy Van Kleunen is Director of Workforce Policy for the Paraprofessional Healthcare Institute. Mary Ann Wilner is the Director of Health Policy at the Paraprofessional Healthcare Institute, Bronx, New York.

Andy Van Kleunen and Mary Ann Wilner can be contacted care of the Paraprofessional Healthcare Institute, 349 East 149th Street, Bronx, NY 10451 (E-mail: maryann@paraprofessional. org).

[Haworth co-indexing entry note]: "Who Will Care for Mother *Tomorrow*?" Kleunen, Andy Van, and Mary Ann Wilner. Co-published simultaneously in *Journal of Aging & Social Policy* (The Haworth Press, Inc.) Vol. 11, No. 2/3, 2000, pp. 115-126; and: *Advancing Aging Policy as the 21st Century Begins* (ed: Francis G. Caro, Robert Morris, and Jill R. Norton) The Haworth Press, Inc., 2000, pp. 115-126. Single or multiple copies of this article are available for a fee from The Haworth Document Delivery Service [1-800-342-9678, 9:00 a.m. - 5:00 p.m. (EST). E-mail address: getinfo@haworthpressinc.com].

care received by long-term care consumers is directly related to the *quality of the job* offered to the paraprofessionals who deliver that care on a day-to-day basis. Creating quality jobs for these frontline workers–who provide 80% to 90% of long-term care service–is thus essential to constructing a high-quality, cost-effective, long-term care delivery system.

Unfortunately, healthcare policymakers have failed to address–or, in many cases, even acknowledge–these frontline issues. As a result, we are in the midst of a growing nationwide shortage of direct care workers available to meet the mounting needs of millions of Americans who are elderly, chronically ill, or living with disabilities (Foltz-Gray, 1997).

To overcome this shortage, we must first understand its causes, and then identify ways to create jobs that are attractive to caregivers–jobs that pay well, provide benefits, offer training and advancement opportunities, and afford respect. To that end, this essay offers a closer look at paraprofessional caregivers and the nature of their jobs, summarizes some of the public policies that currently shape the quality of those jobs, and proposes some possible steps that policymakers could take to start rebuilding our nation's direct-care workforce.

WHO ARE THE PARAPROFESSIONAL CAREGIVERS?

Paraprofessional caregivers are home health aides, certified nursing assistants (CNAs), personal attendants, and other frontline caregivers working in nursing homes, assisted-living facilities, adult-care homes, group homes for the mentally and physically disabled, and individual clients' residences. All told, these workers accounted in 1993 for more than 2.25 million positions, or 20% of our nation's healthcare workforce (Himmelstein, Lewontin, & Woolhandler, 1996).

Over 90% of these paraprofessionals are women, most of them aged 22 to 45. They are also disproportionately women of color–comprising 30% of direct-care workers nationwide, and the majority of paraprofessionals in many urban centers. In fact, one fifth of African-American women employed in the United States work within health care–many of them in direct-care jobs (Himmelstein et al., 1996). Direct-care jobs are also a common source of employment for many recent immigrants.

Finally, many of these low-income women have entered these healthcare jobs after a period of time on public assistance–including individuals who have cycled on and off welfare repeatedly to compensate for intermittent stretches of part-time paraprofessional employment. This pool of potential direct-care workers, as we will discuss later, may be attenuating with recent changes in federal welfare policy.

WHAT ARE THEIR JOBS LIKE?

In exchange for their vital work, CNAs and home health aides earn hourly wages averaging between $6.00 and $7.00 an hour. Annual incomes for CNAs and home health aides range from $11,000 for new workers, to $12,600 (home care), and $14,500 (CNAs) for experienced workers–putting the typical direct-care worker below the poverty line (Marion Merrell Dow, 1995; SEIU, 1997).

Besides low wages, paraprofessional incomes are also suppressed by the limited availability of full-time jobs. Over 70% of home health aides, and more than 30% of CNAs in nursing homes, are able to secure only part-time work–forcing many of them to attempt juggling two or more such jobs simultaneously with different employers (Crown, 1994).

Employer-paid health insurance is also a rarity within most direct care workplaces. This is related, in part, to the prevalence of part-time work. But even many full-time paraprofessionals lack an employer-sponsored health plan–or if such a plan is offered, its premium contributions and co-payments make it too expensive to be used by these low-wage workers.

An increasing, but uncountable, number of home care paraprofessionals delivering personal assistance services are not even "employed" in the typical sense of the word. They are working as "independent providers" hired by individual long-term care consumers, who then pay their caregivers with public Medicaid dollars, private insurance, or their own out-of-pocket cash. Working in such informal settings, these workers have little recourse to Fair Labor Standards Act protections (e.g., minimum wage or overtime pay). They likewise enjoy few, if any, benefits: no health insurance, and often no employer payment into Social Security or state unemployment insurance funds.

Direct care is also literally back-breaking work–particularly, in cases in which caregivers are constantly lifting and moving clients without sufficient equipment or staff assistance. Annually, certified nursing assistants (CNAs) are injured more than workers in mining, construction, or steel mill jobs–and the nursing home industry claims the highest rate of occupational illness and injury of any of the country's 20 fastest-growing employment sectors (Service Employees International Union, 1995).

Training for direct care workers–where mandated at all–is usually short (75 to 100 hours) and often inadequate to help caregivers succeed at their demanding jobs. Many categories of direct-care workers receive no formal training at all, even though they are caring for many of the same types of clients as "trained" paraprofessionals. And there are few opportunities for skill upgrading or advancement for incumbent direct-care workers–thereby limiting their access to career paths or their prospects for long-term employment in the sector.

Finally, direct-care workers lack opportunities for involvement in care planning or other quality-assurance activities even though they are the eyes and ears of the client. All of these conditions contribute to high levels of turnover which destroy the valued relationships upon which caregiving is based.

WHAT IS CAUSING THE WORKER SHORTAGE?

From this brief snapshot of direct-care workers and the conditions of their employment, we can began to sketch a larger picture of why our nation is facing such a mounting paraprofessional labor shortage.

Experienced Caregivers Cannot Earn a Liveable Wage from These Jobs

These positions–which are administered mostly by agencies in the private sector, but are paid for primarily with public Medicare and Medicaid dollars–typically offer poverty-level wages and few benefits. As public health-care budget cuts continue to depress the real wages of these "public employees once removed," even the most committed caregivers are being forced to leave the jobs and the clients they love for better-paying positions outside of health care.

Fewer New Workers Are Entering These Jobs

In today's economy, there are many lower-skilled jobs that pay more and demand less than positions in long-term care. Again, since this is an employment sector in which wage and benefit levels respond primarily to changes in public policy–not shifts in market demand –paraprofessional wages are being outpaced by jobs in other sectors like retail and hospitality. In addition, many of the low-income women who once entered these positions through welfare-to-work job training programs can no longer do so because of new, stringent "work first" policies that do not support pre-employment training like that required by home health aide or CNA certification (see Figure 1). Fewer women comprise the "caregiving workforce."

Many of America's long-term care workers–especially those who work in nursing homes–are women aged 25-44 years. Yet demographic projections indicate that the number of American working women in this age bracket is now *declining* (Foltz-Gray, 1997). Hence, in the decades ahead, we will see an absolute drop in the number of women who might consider becoming a direct-care worker.

FIGURE 1. The Disappearing Worker

Impending Labor Shortages in Paraprofessional Health Care

Americans Age 80 and Over

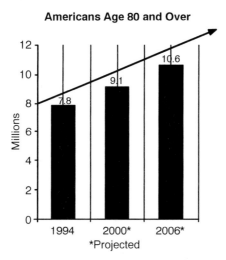

**Women in the U.S. Civilian
Workforce: Aged 25 to 44**

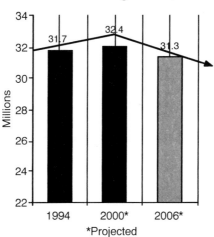

The looming shortage of women aged 25 through 44 in the civilian workforce was first noted by Dorothy Foltz-Gray in an article entitled "The Disappearing Worker," *Contemporary Long Term Care*, October 1997.

Increasing Numbers of People
Are in Need of Long-Term Care

Even as the number of potential caregivers is poised to decrease, the number of people requiring caregiving services–and the intensity of the care requirements of clients who are now living longer–is already growing dramatically, and will continue to do so for decades to come.

THE CURRENT ROLE OF PUBLIC POLICY

Our nation's long-term care delivery system is thus facing a significant worker shortage that is likely to become even more critical in the years ahead. So what are federal policymakers doing to close this ever-widening labor gap and to respond to growing consumer demands for a more stable and experienced direct-care workforce? Unfortunately, a range of current federal policies–from reimbursement and regulatory standards within healthcare policy, to public training programs within welfare and workforce development policy–are only serving to exacerbate the problem.

Healthcare Policy

Despite recent budget cutbacks, federal agencies are still the nation's largest payers for long-term care services through Medicare, Medicaid, Older American Act funds, and Social Service Block Grants. As such, the federal government is the "employer once removed" for millions of direct-care workers. Yet these public agencies–despite their interest in tracking down waste and fraud within their programs–have little knowledge of how tax dollars are actually being used (or not) by private contractors to support frontline workers in their hands-on delivery of long-term care services. For example, the Health Care Finance Administration (HCFA) has never asked home health agencies or nursing homes to report on how much a reimbursement for paraprofessional service goes to agency overhead and profit versus to the wages, benefits, or support of the worker actually delivering that service to her client.

What's more, federal healthcare agencies do not take "labor impact" into account when proposing changes in long-term care policy. While HCFA accompanies any proposed alteration in long-term care reimbursement or regulation with an assessment of the measure's potential impact on providers, consumers, and even the amount of paperwork it might generate, the agency offers no comparable assessment of whether the initiative might lead to lay-offs, wage reductions, or the further destabilization of the workforce expected to deliver those direct care services.

Welfare/Workforce Development Policy

Many paraprofessional workers, especially those in home care, have supplemented their part-time incomes with public supports such as Medicaid, or assistance with childcare payments and transportation costs. During episodes when they had no work because their clients were hospitalized, had been discharged, or had died, they could easily return to public supports. However, now that welfare reform is moving many of these individuals off of welfare, their opportunities to supplement part-time work with public supports have eroded, and these workers are forced to seek full-time work in other sectors.

The healthcare system generally takes responsibility for supporting the training of its professionals (e.g., doctors, nurses), but it has largely left the public support of training for direct-care workers to welfare-to-work or workforce development operations funded by programs like the Job Training Partnership Act, Jobs Opportunities and Basic Skills, and myriad related state and local programs. These programs had helped many low-income adults access healthcare employment by funding their training to become home health aides or CNAs–positions that, according to federal mandate, require pre-employment skill training and certification.

However, since the 1996 passage of "welfare reform," the federal government, and many states receiving federal welfare funds, have drastically curtailed welfare recipients' enrollment in education or skill training, promoting instead a strict "work first" paradigm that emphasizes getting a job–any job–over gaining skills as the means of entry into the workforce. As a result, many low-income adults who would have received training to become a home health or nursing home worker are now being steered by their caseworkers *away* from such direct care positions–precisely because of their pre-employment skill-training requirements.

Ironically, the U.S. Department of Health and Human Services (DHHS)–the agency which houses HCFA where paraprofessional certification standards are set–is also the federal agency implementing welfare reform with training exclusions. As a result, the agency that should be ensuring an adequate supply of direct-care workers is, at the same time, forbidding many potential direct-care workers from receiving the training they need to enter those jobs. Furthermore, DHHS's "labor blind" long-term care policies are doing little to improve the retention levels of those paraprofessional jobs, thereby condemning many low-wage workers to eventually cycle out of these high turnover positions and potentially back onto welfare.

POLICY PRESCRIPTIONS

We believe that federal and state governments–as the primary purchasers and regulators of long-term care services–could use their significant leverage over this sector to effect the changes that could improve the stability and competency of the direct-care workforce and ensure its sufficient size to meet growing consumer demand. Some of the following policy options we propose are budget neutral, requiring only that a portion of current long-term care resources be tracked and earmarked for workforce support and improvement. Other proposals would require new spending–a seemingly untenable option within today's tight budgetary environment, but, when compared to the high costs of staff turnover and instability, an approach that policymakers should seriously consider.

For example, the replacement of a single CNA or home health aide costs between $3,000 and $4,000–a sizeable expense, especially for providers with workforce turnover approaching 100% a year. Agencies that rely on temporary replacement workers to fill these vacancies likewise spend twice what it would normally cost them to pay an in-house caregiver. Even greater–and more shameful–are the costs in care quality that are shifted onto the backs of long-term care clients. Without the benefit of a sufficient number of trained, competent staff, long-term care clients are more prone to become malnourished, dehydrated, incontinent or depressed, and more likely to require expensive medical interventions or hospitalizations when the quality of day-to-day services breaks down.

Hence, we propose that the federal government take the lead in bringing greater public attention to the issues facing direct-care workers, and consider the following steps to improve this vital workforce.

It Should Convene a Federal Inter-Agency Working Group

Many of the policy problems cited above originate from a general lack of attention to direct-care worker issues, and an absence of communication between individual federal agencies that each influence a different aspect of paraprofessional training and job quality. Healthcare officials within DHHS want a better long-term care workforce, but they refuse to see these workers as under their purview, disclaiming any responsibility for the quality of their jobs. Welfare officials within DHHS see many direct-care workers as low-income "clients"–many of them people whom the federal government wants to keep off public assistance; yet these officials know very little about the long-term care industry, in which hundreds of thousands of those clients are so tentatively employed. And workforce development officials within the U.S. Department of Labor–likewise concerned about moving people from welfare to work–currently see direct-care jobs as paying too little and offering too few chances of success to warrant a public investment of job-training dollars.

The goals of these agencies could all be served by a more stable direct-care workforce employed by an industry that offers family-sustaining incomes and benefits, long-term job retention, and ongoing opportunities for skill upgrading. But the public policies needed to achieve those ends will never transpire until these various federal actors agree to come together and treat the direct-care workforce as a shared priority. A federal inter-agency working group would be one important step toward creating that foundation for policy changes. The work group should:

Investigate How Our Long-Term Care Dollars Are Being Spent

As a condition of receiving federal Medicare or Medicaid reimbursement, HCFA should require that long-term care providers report on their frontline workforce's turnover, training, and wages and benefits–and on how public dollars are being used (or not) to achieve those outcomes. This would establish greater accountability from these private agencies, and it would create a baseline from which the government might begin to assess how to improve more broadly the hands-on delivery of these services. Such data could also be shared with consumers–as part of a provider "report card"–so clients and their families could make more informed choices about different providers based on the stability of their direct-care workforce.

Require and Support Better Training

The federal government has set some standards for paraprofessional certification within nursing homes and Medicare home health, but these have proven largely inadequate. Furthermore, entire segments of the direct care workforce, particularly under Medicaid, have no training standards at all. The federal government needs to create better and more uniform training standards across a range of comparable direct-care positions. The federal government should allocate training resources–whether through expansions of targeted healthcare reimbursements, or through the diversion of available welfare and workforce development funds (e.g., customized job training under the Workforce Investment Act, USDOL Welfare-to-Work grants, millions of surplus federal welfare dollars currently sitting in state coffers) toward the training, retention, and upgrading of low-wage healthcare workers.

Successful use of training dollars should be measured by the percentage of workers who remain in the job past six months or a year. We know that a very high percentage of newly recruited workers are likely to leave these jobs in the first 90 days because they are unprepared, emotionally or technically, to meet the job demands. According to Genevieve Gipson, the real test of a successful agency is the proportion of workers who are long-stayers. Identifying what providers can do to foster long-stayers is essential to creating attractive jobs.

Change the Reimbursement Structures

Several state Medicaid programs have used mechanisms like "wage pass-throughs" to ensure that a certain portion of its long-term care payments to agencies are passed on by employers directly to frontline workers. Such initiatives have multiplied over the past year in response to current labor shortages. The federal government should heed the states' example, and consider how to pass along some of its own Medicare/Medicaid dollars to support frontline wages, training, and so forth.

A second consideration should be the variability in reimbursement rates across different programs (Medicare, Medicaid) and settings (home health, personal services, nursing home) for similar services provided by comparably skilled paraprofessionals. For example, differences in wage rates between home care and nursing home positions have put home care clients at even greater risk of not finding a qualified caregiver–primarily because nursing homes have been more proactive in securing additional public resources to attract workers. Rather than pitting long-term care consumers against each other, the federal government should spearhead an effort to promote equity and consistency in wage rates for caregivers across these settings.

Ensure Health Insurance for Healthcare Workers

Through the Children's Health Insurance Program and other initiatives, the federal government has created vehicles to guarantee health coverage for greater numbers of low-income Americans. In addition, some states have expanded coverage for working adults living just above the poverty line–including targeting public health benefits to workers within particular industries that rarely offer employer-paid health insurance (e.g., Rhode Island's childcare workers). The federal government should likewise address the tragic irony of healthcare workers without healthcare coverage through an industry-specific "healthcare for healthcare workers" initiative–a campaign that could significantly reduce paraprofessional turnover and workforce instability.

WHAT ELSE IS NEEDED?

While it is not the focus of this article, we know that policy change alone will not suddenly eradicate paraprofessional turnover or make direct-care work a sustainable career. Changes in industry practice–the ways home care agencies and nursing homes train and supervise direct-care workers, meaningfully involve paraprofessionals in quality-assurance systems, and structure the delivery of paraprofessional services–will likewise be required to substantially improve the quality of direct-care jobs.

Thankfully, some select nursing home and home health agencies have already begun to reorient their management philosophies and practices in this manner, embarking on "replacing the typical low-investment, temporary personnel approach" prevalent throughout the long-term care industry "with a strategy of high investment in frontline employees, emphasizing careful recruitment, decent wages and benefits, full-time work, extensive training, counseling, and support" (Wilner, 1999).

For example, the *Pioneer Movement*–a growing number of nursing homes nurturing cultures emphasizing community and relationships–have involved their CNAs in care planning, decisionmaking, and problem-solving. And the *Cooperative Healthcare Network*–a federation of four worker-owned home care cooperatives that employ more than 600 home health aides–has shown that direct-care jobs can become long-term vehicles of employment and advancement through cooperative ownership, extensive training, and support and advancement opportunities (Wilner & Wyatt, 1998).

Of course, such industry-based innovations have required not only a new perspective on how direct-care workers should be valued and respected. Many of them have also relied on grants or other outside funds not typically leveraged by long-term care providers. As we look toward changing industry practice within long-term care, the issue of public resources thus inevitably resurfaces as a factor in supporting such changes. Again, that may seem unlikely when much of the long-term care industry is already reeling from recent Medicare cuts, and state Medicaid programs are struggling to pick up some of the costs previously shouldered by the federal government. Individual consumers are likewise picking up a larger portion of the long-term care bill–whether through out-of-pocket expenditures or the purchase of long-term care insurance–to pay for services not covered by either Medicare or Medicaid.

But public officials cannot escape the fact that the current workforce shortages will continue to face long-term care providers and consumers for decades to come. In the current full-employment economy, many people are working–they just are not working in direct care. Even if the current economic prosperity subsides, demographics alone point to a gaping hole in our nation's long-term care delivery system. Continued inability to attract, retain, and upgrade our direct care workforce will put at jeopardy the availability of life-preserving services for millions of Americans who are elderly, chronically ill, or living with disabilities. If our federal and state policymakers are not prepared to abdicate responsibility for supporting long-term care in this country, then they will have to wrestle with what investments will be necessary to attract, hold onto, and upgrade our nation's long-term care workforce.

AUTHOR NOTES

Andy Van Kleunen is Director of Workforce Policy for the Paraprofessional Healthcare Institute. He was a graduate fellow in urban sociology at the New School for Social Research. He co-staffs the National Workforce Alliance, a collection of workforce development organizations interested in bringing a practitioner's perspective into federal workforce development and welfare-to-work policymaking. The group also presses for public support of effective practices in community-based training and employment that have helped low-income adults access long-term, living-wage jobs.

Mary Ann Wilner is Director of Health Policy at the Paraprofessional Healthcare Institute, Bronx, New York. She coordinates the Direct Care Alliance, a national, grassroots coalition of consumers, workers, and concerned providers who are dedicated to improving the quality of long-term care through creating better jobs for frontline workers. She also develops and teaches college level courses for home health workers in a collaborative program with Lehman College, City University of New York. The Paraprofessional Healthcare Institute is a national nonprofit healthcare employment development and advocacy organization, based in the South Bronx, that links a network of worker-owned healthcare providers specializing in paraprofessional services. Its mission is to (1) provide high-quality healthcare to clients who are elderly, chronically ill, and disabled, and (2) create decent jobs for low-income women.

REFERENCES

Crown, W.H. (1994, Fall). A national profile of home care, nursing home, and hospital aides. *Generations, XVIII*(3) 29-33.

Foltz-Gray, D. (1997, October). The disappearing worker. *Contemporary Long Term Care*, 62-67.

Himmelstein, D.U., Lewontin, J.P., & Woolhandler, S. (1996, April). Medical care employment in the United States, 1968 to 1993: The importance of health sector jobs for African Americans and women. *American Journal of Public Health, 86*, (4) 525-528.

Marion Merrell Dow. (1995 and 1996). *Managed care digest long term care edition.* Kansas City, MO.

Service Employees International Union, 1995. *Caring till it hurts.* Washington, DC.

Wilner, M.A. (1999, Jan/Feb). On the front lines of healthcare. *Health Progress, 80*(1) 80.

Wilner, M.A., & Wyatt, A. (1998). *Paraprofessionals on the front lines: Improving their jobs–Improving the quality of long-term care: A conference background paper.* Washington, DC: AARP.

Uneasy Allies:
Nursing Home Regulators
and Consumer Advocates

Iris C. Freeman, MSW

Advocacy Center for Long-Term Care
Bloomington, Minnesota

KEYWORDS. Ombudsman, regulation, nursing homes, advocacy

Nursing-home quality problems are destined to outlast the century despite the earnest efforts of dedicated people. This essay focuses on one element of the consumer protection system, the working relationships between nursing home regulators and consumer advocates, particularly advocates in designated ombudsman programs. The proposition is that a fresh lens on their interdependence will surface achievable means to improve the effectiveness of the consumer protection system.

Iris C. Freeman joined the Alzheimer's Association, Minnesota-Lakes Chapter, as Director of Public Policy in January 2000. Previously, she directed the Advocacy Center for Long-Term Care in Bloomington, Minnesota, from 1977 to 1999; she wrote the above essay during that period. Her efforts have included client advocacy, educational materials, and policy initiatives. She served on the Institute of Medicine Committee on Nursing Home Regulation, Washington, D.C., and subsequently as an OBRA Impact Assessment Advisor to the Health Care Financing Administration.

Iris Freeman can be contacted care of the Alzheimer's Association, Minnesota-Lakes Chapter, 4570 West 77th Street, Suite 198, Edina, MN 55435 (E-mail: Iris.Freeman@alz.org).

[Haworth co-indexing entry note]: "Uneasy Allies: Nursing Home Regulators and Consumer Advocates." Freeman, Iris C. Co-published simultaneously in *Journal of Aging & Social Policy* (The Haworth Press, Inc.) Vol. 11, No. 2/3, 2000, pp. 127-135; and: *Advancing Aging Policy as the 21st Century Begins* (ed: Francis G. Caro, Robert Morris, and Jill R. Norton) The Haworth Press, Inc., 2000, pp. 127-135. Single or multiple copies of this article are available for a fee from The Haworth Document Delivery Service [1-800-342-9678, 9:00 a.m. - 5:00 p.m. (EST). E-mail address: getinfo@haworthpressinc.com].

To external observers, it may seem that advocates' relationships with regulators have all the mercurial fluctuations of teenage romances. One day, the advocate is appealing to state officials for regulators' budgets and enforcement authorities with such fervor that some legislators conclude that the agencies are really a single organism. Later that same day, the advocate is on the evening news, standing before a sea of microphones, denouncing regulatory shortcomings. Regulators, in a somewhat less public way, admit to both complimentary and hostile views of the advocates. If there is a method to these dynamics, it is likely an unplanned one.

This essay, written from the consumer advocates' side of the ledger, compares the diverse yet compatible roles of the two entities, identifies existing bases for collaboration, recommends principles for more effective connections, and recognizes that effective relationships alone are insufficient to improve the safety of nursing home consumers. The underlying policy perspectives are these: First, uneasy as the allies may often be, the mission of nursing home consumer protection will continue to require both regulatory and community involvement. Individually, neither office has the authorities nor the resources to respond to the breadth of consumers' inquiries and problems. Even together, the potential for sufficiency is doubtful. Second, there is vulnerability in common. Both regulatory and advocacy practitioners come under fire in the course of their work from legislators and the nursing home industry. Some opponents seem to distinguish between health department surveyors and ombudsmen only to the extent of considering the former to be *official* intermeddlers and the latter *officious* intermeddlers.

DIVERSE AND COMPATIBLE ROLES

State and federal nursing home regulators have a mandate to protect the public's health and safety in nursing homes. There are three components: establishing explicit criteria (standards, markers, rules) to govern nursing home behavior and operations; establishing and carrying out standard methods for monitoring nursing home performance (through periodic facility-wide inspections and individual complaint investigations); and taking enforcement action where unsatisfactory performance is substantiated (Institute of Medicine, 1986, p. 12).

Long-term care ombudsmen, by contrast, operate through a program created in 1975 for active advocacy and representation of consumers. The federal mandate of the Older Americans Act encompasses complaint investigation, volunteer training and deployment, monitoring the development of laws and regulations that affect nursing home consumers, and informing public agencies about the problems consumers experience in long-term care. To strengthen that capacity, the most recent amendments to the Older Americans Act, enacted in 1987 and 1992, instructed states to assure ombudsmen access to residents and their records, and gave them other legal protections. States have considerable flexibility in designing their programs; however, each program is expected to yield the foregoing range of services. The ombudsman program's keystone is personal attention to residents as a means to overcome the inherent limitations of regulatory approaches (Institute of Medicine, 1995, pp. 42-45).

BASES FOR COLLABORATION

Since the mid-1980s, nursing home consumer-protection studies have recommended linkage between nursing home regulatory agencies and external advocacy organizations. The Institute of Medicine Committee on Nursing Home Regulation, in its 1986 report, *Improving the Quality of Care in Nursing Homes*, recommended that the Health Care Financing Administration require states to make public all nursing home inspection and cost reports. The panel advised that these documents be readily accessible at nominal cost to consumers and consumer advocates, including state and local ombudsmen. The orientation of this recommendation was that regulators' time at a facility is inherently brief and focused. Ombudsmen and consumer advocates, adequately informed of findings, have the opportunity and the incentive to track facilities' responses over time, watchful that successes be sustained and problems be corrected.

By 1995, the Institute of Medicine's study of the Long-term Care Ombudsman Program illustrated that the working relationship already extended far beyond sharing reports. Long-term care ombudsman programs, yeomen of the regulatory reform effort, were

> active in advocating for changes, monitoring the conduct of regulatory reform, providing training and consultation to state surveyors and the staff at individual facilities on quality of life and rights issues, training at the individual facility level, and informing residents and families about the reform. (Institute of Medicine, 1995, p. 38)

Significant integration toward direct involvement of nursing home ombudsmen staff and volunteers in preparation for nursing home surveys and survey exit conferences had come with the enactment of the Nursing Home Reform Law of 1987 (PL 100-203). The operations manual for state surveyors now expressly directs that offsite survey preparation include this task:

> Contact the ombudsman office in accordance with the policy developed between the State survey agency and the State ombudsman agency. The

purposes of this contact are to notify the ombudsman of the proposed day of entrance into the facility and to obtain any information the ombudsman wishes to share with the survey team. Ask if the ombudsman will be available if the residents participating in the group or individual interviews wish her/him to be present. (HCFA, Survey Procedures for Long-Term Care Facilities, 1995, p. P-5)

At the close of the inspection, surveyors are directed to invite the ombudsman to the exit conference at the facility (p. P-46). On the tangible level, coordination is directed. On the symbolic level, this change in the survey process deemed representatives of the ombudsman program "insiders" enough to be privy to otherwise highly guarded information.

A subsequent state-level study in Oregon examined the relationship between ombudsman activities and enforcement actions by nursing home regulatory agencies. Oregon ombudsmen, like others around the country, have firsthand responsibility for the bulk of conflict resolution, and refer certain categories of suspected abuse to adult protective service and nursing home regulatory agencies. Often, the situations referred are those that might have gone unnoticed and unreported without the ombudsman presence. The study authors' hypotheses were that ombudsman activity would promote abuse complaints and substantiated findings, sanction activity, and survey deficiencies. Results did support the increased abuse complaints and substantiation; however, abuse investigations are performed by adult protective services rather than the nursing home licensing agency. With respect to sanctions and survey deficiencies, there were connections if not causality, and the authors concluded that "regulatory agency activity is significantly greater in nursing facilities with ombudsmen" than those without (Nelson, Huber, & Walter, 1995).

Four years later, the Report of the Office of Inspector General on the overall capacity of the Ombudsman Program carried forward the principle that the "ombudsman program is distinct from and complements other nursing home monitoring programs" and vice versa. Its analysis is that ombudsman program capacity is enhanced by collaboration with other monitoring programs. Then, citing this level of collaboration in just 61% of nursing home surveys in 1997, the Report concluded with a recommendation that the Administration on Aging take the lead in helping states enhance collaboration between ombudsman and survey and certification agencies (Office of the Inspector General, 1999a).

March 1999 saw the publication of another report from the Office of the Inspector General. This one focused on the deficiency trends documented by nursing home survey and certification agencies. With findings of chronic problems in some facilities and identified systemic weaknesses in the survey process, these OIG recommendations also direct surveyors to facilitate better coordination with the Ombudsman Program (Office of the Inspector General, 1999b).

Amid this uniform message, it should be noted that these productive ties have to recognize boundaries, because some connections are ill-advised, even prohibited. For compliance with the Older Americans Act, a nursing home ombudsman program must not be part of an entity that is responsible for licensing or certifying long-term care facilities. To do so constitutes a conflict of interest (Institute of Medicine, 1995, p. 103).

PRINCIPLES FOR CONNECTION

Beyond the stipulated synergy in the survey process, the Institute of Medicine (1995, p. 181) identified among exemplary ombudsman practices an ongoing interaction with regulatory agencies that includes discussing plans for future actions at "pre-decision points," and planning and carrying on joint trainings, with approaches that make the most of each partner's strength. In a nutshell, the goal envisions both premeditation and spontaneity, joint ventures and those that are necessarily singular, with the recognition that regulators regulate and advocates (the noun) advocate (the verb). The following are three principles for these effective, elastic connections.

Join Forces for Survival

A generation of nursing home reform activity at state and national levels is marked by the advocacy for a public health approach to nursing home performance. To the extent that regulators are limited by the agencies' protocols, advocates have had to represent nursing home inspectors who are, in the legislative budgeting process, as voiceless as the residents. In a similar vein, consumer representatives are typically alone in challenging state budgetary cutbacks for nursing home surveys or complaint inspections, and they are alone at the microphone when there is a need to support enforcement authority. In 1997, Minnesota advocates successfully sought new state funds to replace what the State Health Department's Office of Health Facility Complaints had accounted as lost in three successive years of federal budget cuts. While these funds were a priority initiative for the advocates, the State Health Commissioner had sought no new state funds for long-term care regulation. Consumer advocates provided legislators with questions to promote analysis of the Department budget's adequacy as well as questions about the stability of federal funds, the potential of carryover state funds from the current budget period, vacancies in the workforce for nursing home inspections and complaint investigations, backlogs in complaint investigations, and Department policies that curtailed certain categories of complaint investigations, for example, on residents' rights cases. Later, as opportunities arose for public testimony on Departmental budgets, these issues were raised and illustrated with case examples from the ombudsman program. Of the $430,000 federal dollars lost, $402,000 were restored in state support. One might assume that the corollary for occupying the same side of the fence is that regulatory agencies will be counted on to raise a flag or a ruckus when ombudsman programs are similarly endangered or cut short. That equitable thought is hampered by the reality that overt advocacy may, realistically, exceed the range of motion of regulatory agencies. Nonetheless, the principle of reciprocity, in whatever subtle form, deserves exploration.

Commit to Education

Education is the common ground in the mandates of ombudsman and regulatory offices. Provider education, consumer education, and orientation of one anothers' staffs afford a wide spectrum of opportunities to initiate, plan, and communicate. Another Minnesota example is the production of a pamphlet to improve the comfort level and competencies of nursing home residents and their families within the inspection process. The 1987 Nursing Home Reform Law directed nursing home regulators to interview residents and families in the course of the survey. But the inhibiting effects of the nursing home environment, the unfamiliarity of the rules, and the awkwardness between regulators and consumers were confounding factors. To influence the process, the Minnesota Department of Health contracted with local advocates to produce *Nursing and Boarding Care Home Inspections: Information for Residents, Families, and Visitors*. This large-type booklet described the survey process from the residents' point of view, introduced the interview process and how consumers could be involved, identified some of the issues surveyors would raise, offered advice about fears of retaliation for identifying negative aspects of life in the home, discussed how surveyors inspect for the intangibles related to the quality of life, and provided a glossary of terms about public regulation and consumer protection. Without the Department of Health's request for proposal and funding, the booklet might not have been written or distributed. Without the consumer organization's design and plain language, the booklet might not have been as well-suited to its audience. It was a good match, although ad hoc and comparatively spontaneous. A better approach in the future, applicable in any jurisdiction, would be to build an educational agenda through an annual joint review of survey and complaint office results as well as ombudsman casework.

Fight Fairly, but Fight

As the title of this essay implies, the relationship is not an endless chorus of chummy summer camp songs. Few aspects of ombudsman casework are more frustrating than recognizing that advising a nursing home resident or family member to notify the Department of Health may result in neither investigation nor redress.

Client advocacy implicitly involves intervening with a public agency on a client's behalf. Client advocacy with nursing home regulators on behalf of nursing home residents and their families too often feels like a collision with a brick wall. The messages conveyed by the regulator to the advocate are these: "That situation is not enough of an emergency." "That case happened too long ago." "You are misreading the law; there is nothing unlawful to investigate."

Regarding the emergency status of a case referral, one can accept the fact that any agency apportions its work by setting priorities; however, when broad bands of casework fall outside the articulated priorities or so low on the scale that investigation will not occur at all, the question of accountability must be raised by advocates, and friction is a by-product.

Forbearance of the state agency's shortcomings is tantamount to acceptance that below a certain threshold, as for example a case of residents' privacy in bathing or toileting, there is nowhere to turn for enforcement of nursing home regulations. An ultimate casework breakdown is the juncture where the advocate cannot, and the regulator will not, *order* the nursing home to change its behavior or risk sanction. Residents and families lose hope and trust in both agencies.

On this theme, one is left pondering whether to yearn for the future or for the past. In the past, there was the groundbreaking *Smith* case, in actuality more than a dozen years' series of events aimed at securing regulatory protection for Medicaid recipients in nursing homes. In 1975, a Colorado nursing home resident, Michael Smith, sued his state health agency and the then Department of Health, Education and Welfare for their failure to enforce standards for quality care. This complex and multi-phased case is notable especially for the turn of events in which the state agency leadership came to agree that their program's beneficiaries were ill-served, and thus they moved to the side of the plaintiff to advocate a stronger federal presence in nursing home enforcement. The objectives of the *Smith* case, including uniform resident assessment, a well-honed survey process, and clear standards for effective remedies, are the core of the reforms a decade later.

Challenge in the cause of accountability is a service that can be delivered in a bipartisan manner. Nursing home regulators can and ought to challenge advocates' interpretations, priorities, and understanding of the "big picture." Realistically, the success of such honest conflict rides on the strength of an ongoing relationship, in a spirit of support and respect.

NECESSARY BUT NOT SUFFICIENT

Were the foregoing elements of coordination to be achieved nationwide, long-term care consumer protection would arguably retain serious gaps and flaws in attaining its mission of overall improvement in care. The protagonists would make the most of what they have and likely enjoy improved morale. Measures of effectiveness would be positive, but the degree to which these changes alone would result in safer and more harmonious facilities rates a probable "no" with some notes about a corollary agenda.

The will and the way are not in balance. In 1998, Senate hearings and Presidential initiatives promised sturdy new enforcement tools for State Health Departments. In March 1999, there were reports from the U.S. Department of Health and Human Services Office of the Inspector General, referenced earlier, and the General Accounting Office (GAO) further documenting needs and identifying solutions (GAO, 1999). Cumulatively, the impact of implementation should be a faster schedule of revisits to facilities with deficiencies, quicker response time on complaint investigations, stronger focus on facilities with the weakest records, amplified fines, and better data management in survey agencies.

In childrens' stories and fables, love might be enough to "make it real," but not in nursing home inspections. Sincere words and implementation plans ultimately require a budget and personnel to make them real, including attention to the less obvious budgetary impacts of these changes. When standards, especially enforcement standards, are stengthened, facilities and individuals have more to lose if sanctioned. Therefore, the time and dollar costs of reconsiderations and appeals draw down the base budgets that health inspectors will apply to implementation of the changes.

Like the surveyors, the ombudsmen are strapped. The Institute of Medicine's 1995 evaluation of the program identified the inadequacy of its resources vis-à-vis its mandate, saying that the "full intent of Congress with respect to the state long-term care ombudsman program has not been met in all–indeed, perhaps in not any, state of the union" (Institute of Medicine, p. 185). The Institute of Medicine Committee went on to recommend a ratio of one full-time staff ombudsman for each 2,000 beds, a state funding allocation formula, a requirement for state matching funds, and an audit to prevent excessive use of ombudsman program resources for their host agency's administrative costs. Nevertheless, reauthorization of the Older Americans Act has been stymied since 1995, and the ombudsman program is more certain to face proposed losses than gains in budget and authority in the near future.

With each passing study, the awareness is heightened, and the resources remain stagnant. We approach the next century with chants of "smaller government" at both the state and national levels, while philanthropies are not racing to fund consumer-protection initiatives in long-term care. To break the cycle of periodic scandals followed by Executive initiatives and somber studies, there will have to be a much more critical public dialogue about consumer protection in long-term care, more of a community development approach to problems and solutions. One can speculate, or dare to dream, that the people who call for smaller government are also people who would be appalled to read the case log of unassigned or uninvestigated nursing home complaints documented by the GAO in its 1999 report.

Well beyond the scope of this essay but integral to the mission of consumer protection are the issues of workforce development, training, and compensation; issues of housing for mid- and lower-income seniors; and resolving the patchwork of inconsistent requirements among long-term care services (home care, assisted living, and nursing home) for people with comparable vulnerabilities.

CONCLUSION

To the focal issue of this piece, nursing home regulators and advocates should continue to be uneasy allies. The presence of harmony and periodic conflict can be viewed as a necessary equilibrium rather than weakness. Were the two of us too close, there would be no challenge or discourse about how best to reach goals of safety, quality of care, and comfortable living arrangements for vulnerable adults in long-term care facilities. And if we were too far apart, we would never argue at all.

REFERENCES

Institute of Medicine. (1986). *Improving the quality of care in nursing homes.* Washington, DC: National Academy Press.

Institute of Medicine. (1995). *Real people, real problems: An evaluation of the long-term care ombudsman program of the Older Americans Act.* Washington, DC: National Academy Press.

Nelson, H. W., Huber, R., & Walter, K. L. (1995). The relationship between volunteer long-term care ombudsman and regulatory nursing home actions. *The Gerontologist, 35,* 509-514.

U.S. Department of Health and Human Services Health Care Financing Administration (1995). *Survey protocol for long-term care facilities.* Washington, DC

U.S. Department of Health and Human Services Office of Inspector General (1999a). *Long-term care ombudsman program: Overall capacity.* OEI-02-98-00351. Washington, DC.

U.S. Department of Health and Human Services Office of Inspector General (1999b). *Nursing home survey and certification: Deficiency trends.* OEI-02-98-00331. Washington, DC.

U.S. General Accounting Office (1999). *Complaint investigation processes often inadequate to protect residents.* GAO/HEHS-99-80. Washington, DC.

END OF LIFE

The Future of Physician-Assisted Suicide

Amy Hutchinson, MS

*Florida State University and
Economic Research Services, Inc.
Tallahassee, Florida*

Henry R. Glick, PhD

*Florida State University
Tallahassee, Florida*

KEYWORDS. Autonomy, right to die, physician-assisted suicide, euthanasia

Physician-Assisted Suicide (PAS)[1] is the most recent issue in the long running political conflict in the United States over the right to die. At the core

Amy Hutchinson is Research Associate for Economic Research Services, Inc. She can be contacted care of Economic Research Services, Inc., 4901 Tower Court, Tallahassee, FL 32303 (E-mail: ahutch@ersnet.com). Henry R. Glick is Professor of Political Science, and Research Associate in the Pepper Institute on Aging and Public Policy at Florida State University. He can be contacted care of the Department of Political Science, Box 2230, Florida State University, Tallahassee, FL 32306-2230 (E-mail: hglick@garnet.acns.fsu.edu).

[Haworth co-indexing entry note]: "The Future of Physician-Assisted Suicide." Hutchinson, Amy, and Henry R. Glick. Co-published simultaneously in *Journal of Aging & Social Policy* (The Haworth Press, Inc.) Vol. 11, No. 2/3, 2000, pp. 137-144; and: *Advancing Aging Policy as the 21st Century Begins* (ed: Francis G. Caro, Robert Morris, and Jill R. Norton) The Haworth Press, Inc., 2000, pp. 137-144. Single or multiple copies of this article are available for a fee from The Haworth Document Delivery Service [1-800-342-9678, 9:00 a.m. - 5:00 p.m. (EST). E-mail address: getinfo@haworthpressinc.com].

of this conflict is who has the right to determine when we may die: *us*, as individuals with control over our own bodies and destiny, or *others*, as the medical community or state and federal governments, that claim a public interest in protecting life? Despite some public support, PAS has had little success in judicial and legislative venues. In this article, we summarize the rise of PAS on the national agenda, followed by an examination of its future as a right-to-die policy alternative. The factors that have contributed to very limited official support of PAS are linked to its future in the United States.

THE DEVELOPMENT OF PAS

The recent momentum of PAS began in 1987 with the California Bar Association's endorsement. That same year the Hemlock Society began a California campaign for PAS in a referendum, which failed in 1988 by a small majority. However, the first event to capture national attention was Dr. Jack Kevorkian's first assisted suicide involving Janet Adkins in June 1990. The importance of this focusing event cannot be overstated. Kevorkian's actions vastly widened the scope of this issue so that during 1990 and beyond, over half of all right-to-die coverage in *The New York Times* has focused on assisted suicide. Furthermore, most mass and professional media publications experienced sharp peaks in assisted suicide coverage in 1993 and 1996, the two years in which Kevorkian assisted in the greatest number of suicides–in 1993, 12 and in 1996, 19.[2]

While Kevorkian's actions captured the attention of the general public, he was dismissed as an aberration by most in the medical community. Not until 1991, when an article by Dr. Timothy Quill describing his PAS experience with a long-term patient appeared in the *New England Journal of Medicine*, did PAS command serious consideration by physicians. Within one year, the percentage of medical journal articles on the right-to-die that focused on PAS nearly doubled, from 18% to 29%. PAS continued building momentum when in 1992 Derek Humphry published his best-selling suicide how-to book, *Final Exit*.

Despite increasing attention to PAS, efforts to transform advocacy into policy have mostly been unsuccessful. As in California, a PAS referendum in Washington state failed by a small majority. In 1994, PAS reached a state supreme court for the first time. Following years of legal conflict surrounding Dr. Kevorkian's controversial role, the Michigan Supreme Court ruled that common law supported a ban on PAS. But that same year Oregon voters legalized PAS in a referendum. Legal challenges and a referendum in 1997 were sponsored by opponents in an attempt to repeal the law, but Oregon's Death with Dignity Act became legal in October, 1997. Thus far Oregon is the only state to sanction PAS, whereas 38 states–14 since 1990–have specifically legislated against physician- or other-assisted suicide.

In June 1997, PAS reached the U.S. Supreme Court, but the justices rejected claims to a constitutional right to PAS for the terminally ill (*Washington v. Glucksberg*, No. 96-110 and *Vacco v. Quill*, No. 95-1858). Just weeks later, a similar decision was announced by the Florida Supreme Court. Then, in 1998, 70% of the voters in Dr. Kevorkian's home state of Michigan rejected PAS.

Like the U.S. Supreme Court, the Congress has rarely addressed right-to-die issues, but in June 1998, the Lethal Drug Abuse Prevention Act was introduced into the House and Senate to make PAS illegal nationwide. However, the Congressional session ended before either chamber voted on the proposal. The culmination of the PAS news events occurred in March 1999 when, after a very highly publicized act of voluntary active euthanasia was broadcast on the CBS news program *60 Minutes*, Dr. Jack Kevorkian was convicted of second-degree murder and later sentenced to 10 to 25 years in prison. The most vocal and widely reported advocate of PAS was stopped and silenced. Three months later, the newly proposed Pain Relief Promotion Act, designed to prevent PAS, was introduced in the U.S. House and Senate. As of this writing, one House committee has voted in favor of the new law.

THE FUTURE OF PAS

Unlike previous right-to-die issues and policy proposals, which had been on the public agenda for many decades before gaining widespread popular support and judicial and legislative acceptance, PAS reached the U.S. Supreme Court just 10 years following the California Bar Association's endorsement. It also took only one decade after the first state referendum for the U.S. House and Senate to introduce legislation to ban it.

How did this issue rise from relative obscurity to national prominence in such a short period of time? There are two likely explanations. First, PAS is an outgrowth of right-to-die issues that have been reported very heavily in the mass media since the mid-1960s. In addition, Dr. Kevorkian's early and startling actions served as focusing events which captured enormous media attention. The outgrowth of PAS from earlier right-to-die issues suggests that previous agenda-setting is a powerful stimulant for gaining attention to new issues that emerge from experience with the old. In Kingdon's terms (1995), previous right-to-die innovation had "softened up" the public and made it easier for PAS to win attention. However, Oregon's acceptance of this still nationally controversial policy and Dr. Kevorkian's unstoppable acts also may have led courts and legislatures to take up the issue quickly in order to prevent the possible further adoption of policies favorable to PAS. Recall, too, that most states, other than California, Oregon, Washington, and a few others, are politically and socially conservative, so that banning PAS is a relatively easy legislative hurdle.

Given its minimal success thus far, what is the future of PAS? We speculate that PAS is not likely to be widely legalized in the near future for several reasons, including conflicting public opinion, a generally negative public image, conflict among PAS supporters, continuing well-organized and respected interest-group opposition, and increasing emphasis on alternative policies, primarily regarding palliative care and hospice care.

Public support for PAS at the national level has increased since 1990, but it still is not strongly positive. From 1990 through 1997, national public opinion has fluctuated between a low of 43% in favor in 1992 and a high of 69% favorable in 1997, but slight differences in the wording of survey questions produce widely varying levels of support.[3] Support for PAS has not reached the near unanimous levels of public endorsement for permitting the withdrawal and withholding of treatment from the terminally ill that existed during the 1980s when most of the states enacted living-will laws.

Support for PAS within the medical community is also not high. A 1996 study drawn from the files of the American Medical Association indicates that 36% of the physician respondents would assist in a suicide if it were legal and 24% would participate in euthanasia (Meier, Emmons, Wallenstein, Quill, Morrison, & Cassel, 1998). In studies by Ezekiel J. Emanuel, an oncologist and medical ethicist at the National Institutes of Health, 46% of oncologists supported PAS for the terminally ill in 1994, while only 22% favored it in 1998 (Ezekiel, 1999). Previous experience with the right to die indicates that legislators are unlikely to support PAS until a very large majority of constituents is in favor of it and until other political venues, particularly the courts, have taken the matter under their jurisdiction and given their assent, both of which seem unlikely.

Fluctuating public opinion is linked to the various and often conflicting images of a policy portrayed by the mass media. A positive image links PAS to earlier and well-established medical and right-to-die policies, such as living wills and "do-not-resuscitate" orders, which emphasize patients' dignity, individual rights, and autonomy. A negative image of PAS is framed in terms of involuntary active euthanasia, in which doctors put patients to death without their knowledge or consent. Opponents believe that PAS is contrary to the healing mission of physicians, and requires them to take a much more active role in hastening death than previous policies calling for the withdrawal of fruitless treatment. This negative image was reinforced by the *60 Minutes* program in which Dr. Kevorkian apparently crossed the line from PAS into voluntary active euthanasia for a patient who, at least some will argue, showed second thoughts.

Assessing the tone of media reporting is a way to determine which image of PAS is dominant in the mass agenda (Baumgartner & Jones, 1993). An analysis of the titles of PAS articles reported in the *Reader's Guide to Periodic Literature* indicates that PAS has a long way to go before it is portrayed mostly in a positive way.[4] In 1990, PAS received no positive reports. Since 1992, however, PAS has been treated more favorably, with negative reporting decreasing sharply since 1994. Nevertheless, negative reporting is being replaced more by a neutral rather than a positive tone. Since the public is likely to take cues on unfamiliar issues from the media, media coverage on PAS probably contributes to the oscillation of public opinion.

In addition to wavering public opinion and varied media portrayals, dissension within the ranks of PAS supporters has no doubt hindered legislative success. For example, some of the leading supporters of PAS, among them Dr. Timothy Quill, have questioned the safeguards enacted as part of the Oregon law. They question the desirability of the 15-day waiting period, which they claim may burden some patients who are suffering intolerable pain and are near the point of death. In contrast to the less restrictive provisions supported by Quill and others, Compassion in Dying, a national interest group supporting PAS, would limit the potential effectiveness of PAS laws by calling for the approval of all members of the patient's immediate family (Kamisar, 1998). Agenda-setting theory stresses the importance of unity within groups of interest. Therefore, these types of disagreements reinforce the difficulty in crafting legislation that provides for patient autonomy, while safeguarding against the threat of coercion.

Disagreement among the supporters of PAS, who also are at the margins politically, stands in stark contrast to the mostly unified and powerful PAS opponents. In each of the four states that have held referenda, opposition came from large, experienced, well-funded and highly regarded, high-status organizations: the Catholic Church and the American Medical Association, acting in concert with their state affiliates. Although their reasons for opposition vary, their goal of keeping PAS illegal is the same. The national coordination and unity within these opposition groups, which together reflect substantial mass and professional constituent interests, usually overwhelms and exploits the divisions among PAS supporters. Thus, from a legislator's standpoint, it is far easier to make PAS illegal than to do otherwise. Indeed, the power of these well-established groups in state legislatures probably led PAS supporters to the referendum as ways of avoiding established influential institutions and individuals, and enacting law by appealing directly to the voters.

The final factor that may derail the legality of PAS, at least in the immediate future, is a new focus on attractive policy alternatives, particularly improved palliative care and hospice care. It is the fear of a protracted and painful death that draws many supporters toward PAS as an option, and throughout this national debate, PAS opponents have argued that proper palliative care would negate any need for PAS or euthanasia. In addition, supporters of the hospice movement argue that its interventions to support dying patients will help reduce the desire and demand for assisted suicide. The American Medical Association has developed a new criteria and protocols for caring for dying patients, and medical schools have focused increased emphasis on pain management and end-of-life care. The National Institutes of Health have designated millions of dollars for research on improvements in palliative care. Choice in Dying, the most prominent right-to-die advocacy and information organization, neither endorses nor opposes PAS, but it strongly supports increased attention to palliative care. Even the 1999 version of the Congressional bill making PAS illegal is titled the *Pain Relief Promotion Act.*

If increasing attention to pain management and other attractive substituted policies continues (see Kingdon, 1995), PAS may fade as a likely policy alternative for the right to die. However, a study of the first patients to utilize Oregon's Death with Dignity Act finds that the fear of losing autonomy, not the fear of pain, motivated most of them to request aid in dying (Chin, Hedberg, Higginson, & Fleming, 1999). Additional experience from Oregon may recast this latest right-to-die issue yet again, for even though PAS may disappear for a time from the national political agenda, the problems faced by many terminally ill patients may not be solved through new emphasis on palliative treatment, and finding other ways to end suffering at the end of life may be in high demand once more.

CONCLUSION

PAS is unlikely to become widespread law any time soon. Although public support is gaining, it is not consistent, and well-organized opponents are able to stymie legalization. Also, courts have not supported a right to assisted suicide. However, we speculate that social conditions, as well as the current practice of medicine, will make PAS more attractive. First, Dr. Kevorkian and his assisted suicides will fade as current events, and media coverage probably will become more neutral or even more positive toward PAS. Various prominent right-to-die organizations, particularly Choice in Dying, now are equivocal regarding assisted suicide. It abhors Dr. Kevorkian and fears the rough, impersonal suicide-on-demand image that he created. However, Choice also is sympathetic and respectful of members and others who see the need for PAS, and it continues to call for discussion, that is, to keep the issue on the agenda. The Hemlock Society continues to maintain that PAS should be an option available to the dying. With more favorable press treatment of events and policy discussions, public support for PAS also may become stronger and more steady. Finally, if a state supreme court should grant the right to assisted suicide, policy change could occur very rapidly.

Continued experience with problems facing dying patients also may reinforce PAS. First, legally permissible alternatives for the terminally ill often do not work well. Various research reveals that, despite living will and other laws, many physicians ignore patients' treatment wishes at the end of life, whether those wishes are contained in written documents or communicated orally. Moreover, living wills and other documents are not applicable to various chronic, devastating, and fatal illnesses, such as Lou Gehrig's and other wasting diseases, or they are not invoked or heeded until a patient is on the verge of death. Although advocates of the right to die will continue to seek improvements in physician-patient communication and compliance with living wills, problems will remain. Second, while PAS opponents maintain that effective hospice and palliative care *can* eliminate the need or desire for suicide, there is no evidence that widespread changes have taken place or will have a substantial impact soon on these fields. Consequently, the failure of previous innovations and policy alternatives to solve the end-of-life treatment dilemma may put PAS more prominently on the social agenda once again.

NOTES

1. We distinguish Physician-Assisted Suicide (PAS) from voluntary active euthanasia in which the physician, at the patient's request, directly causes the death of a patient. In PAS, the physician only provides the means by which the patient may commit suicide, such as a prescription of a lethal narcotic.

2. This research begins in 1987 and ends in 1996. The sources of the data for tracking the mass and professional agenda include counts of articles in the following indices: *Reader's Guide to Periodic Literature* and *The New York Times*, for the mass media; and *Index Medicus*, the *Religion Index*, the *Catholic Index, Index to Legal Periodicals*, the *Humanities Index* and the *Social Science Index*, for the professional media.

3. Questions were analyzed from national surveys reported in the *American Public Opinion Index*. The questions for each year are similarly structured, but not identical.

4. Our previous research covered all PAS articles from 1990 to 1996. Following Baumgartner and Jones (1993), we have coded story titles according to whether a proponent of PAS would be happy or unhappy with the title of the article.

AUTHOR NOTES

Amy Hutchison is Research Associate for Economic Research Services, Inc. (ERS) located in Tallahassee, FL. ERS is a professional research firm providing a variety of services in economic and statistical analysis. She is also a doctoral candidate in Political Science at Florida State University.

Henry R. Glick is Professor of Political Science at Florida State University. He teaches and does research on state court systems and judicial policy, including recent work on the right to die. He has authored numerous books and journal articles on the courts and judicial process, and on right to die policy, including *The Right to Die* (Columbia University Press, 1992).

REFERENCES

American Public Opinion Index. (1987-1997). Bethesda, MD: Opinion Research Service.

Baumgartner, F.R., & Jones, B.D. (1993). *Agendas and instability in American politics*. Chicago: University of Chicago Press.

Chin, A.E., Hedberg, K., Higginson, G.K., & Fleming, D.W. (1999, Feb. 18). Legalized physician-assisted suicide in Oregon–The first year's experience. *The New England Journal of Medicine, 340*(7), 577-583.

Emanuel, E.J. (1999, May 17). The end of euthanasia? Death's door. *The New Republic, 220*(20), 15-16.

Famisar, Y. (1998, July). The future of physician-assisted suicide. *Trial*, 48-53.

Kingdon, J.W. (1995). *Agendas, alternatives, and public policies* (2nd Edition). New York: Harper Collins.

Meier, D.E., Emmons, C., Wallenstein, S., Quill, T., Morrison, R.S. & Cassel, C.K. (1998, April 23). A national survey of physician-assisted suicide and euthanasia in the United States. *New England Journal of Medicine, 338*(17), 1193-1201.

Vacco v. Quill. 117 S. Ct. 2293 (1997).

Washington v. Glucksberg. 117 S. Ct. 2302 (1997).

Dying and Social Policy
in the New Millennium

D. Dixon Sutherland, PhD

Stetson University
DeLand, Florida

Rebecca C. Morgan, JD

Stetson University College of Law
St. Petersburg, Florida

KEYWORDS. Brain death, end-of-life decisionmaking, hospices, palliative care, futility, religion and dying, ethical dilemmas, persistent vegetative state

Used to be that the gauge for successful health care was measured by the question: "How old may we grow?" The "health" of health care rested on number of years lived. An aging population facing the new millennium is refocusing the question. The interest is no longer simply how long, but rather, *"How* may we grow old?" Health concerns have shifted from the span of

---

D. Dixon Sutherland is Professor of Religious Studies and Director of the Institute for Christian Ethics at Stetson University. Address correspondence to: Dixon Sutherland, Professor of Religious Studies, Stetson University, DeLand, FL 32720 (E-mail: dsutherl@stetson.edu). Rebecca C. Morgan is Professor of Law at Stetson University College of Law and Director of the Center for Law and Aging. Address correspondence to: Rebecca Morgan, Stetson University College of Law, 1401 61st Street, St. Petersburg, FL 33707 (E-mail: morgan@hermes.law.stetson.edu).

[Haworth co-indexing entry note]: "Dying and Social Policy in the New Millennium." Sutherland, D. Dixon, and Rebecca C. Morgan. Co-published simultaneously in *Journal of Aging & Social Policy* (The Haworth Press, Inc.) Vol. 11, No. 2/3, 2000, pp. 145-155; and: *Advancing Aging Policy as the 21st Century Begins* (ed: Francis G. Caro, Robert Morris, and Jill R. Norton) The Haworth Press, Inc., 2000, pp. 145-155. Single or multiple copies of this article are available for a fee from The Haworth Document Delivery Service [1-800-342-9678, 9:00 a.m. - 5:00 p.m. (EST). E-mail address: getinfo@haworthpressinc.com].

145

years to quality of life. The major concerns, especially for the elderly, gravitate around how growing old proceeds. When it comes to length of life, the most important concern is not quantity but quality. In this essay, we offer our opinions on the causes, the issues, and the failure to implement an effective decisionmaking process outside of the courts, and conclude with a call for societal institutions to take a leadership role in resolution.

Why this shift? Of course, the fundamental cause is technology. The last half century has undoubtedly seen history's greatest developments in medical technology. These advancements in knowledge and know-how have resulted in abilities to save and extend life in extraordinary ways. End-of-life decisionmaking therefore becomes much more complicated. In a short 50 years, we have moved from determining death by "the foggy mirror" to staving off death by using ventilators, respirators, gastrostomy tubes, and myriad other monitoring agents, and to using brain death as a criterion. To use a biological analogy, when it comes to determination of death, we have moved from breath to brain.

The purpose of all these technological capabilities is to save and extend life, even in the worst circumstances. Running parallel to these capabilities and their usage has been the assumption that *if* a technological ability is available, *then* it must be used. Medical science has thus pushed the limits of death back further and further, until a body can be biologically maintained long after any hope of recovery of the person has faded. Humans may now enter the dark exile of what medicine commonly refers to as PVS, persistent (or permanent) vegetative state. We should not miss the irony of our collective societal circumstance. Advances in medical treatments that highlight the end of this century ironically call forth challenges for the next: How do we as a society fairly and justly develop the ability *not to use or to withdraw* all the technological capabilities we have gained during the last part of the century? Of course, our guide for this stark challenge has already been marked with the *Quinlan* case in 1975, followed by those of Paul Brophy, Nancy Cruzan, and many others. While most people are not aware of the intricacies of the legal battles encircling these issues, they are clearly cognizant of the resulting symbolic phrase, a phrase that embodies what most Americans claim as their right–"the right to die." But the issues of withholding or withdrawing medical treatment are not at all settled. Questions of guardianship, confusion over the authority of advance directives, limits to physician obligations to patients, limits to patient autonomy, and the role of private and societal economics continue to cause serious tensions in end-of-life decisionmaking.

Still, there is more. These very public battles over such personal matters touched a nerve in the psyche of Americans, especially the elderly. For them the focus of the "right to die" is really the right to reject the potential meaningless prolongation of a biological existence without consciousness or function, a possibility now made more likely than ever. On the other extreme, utilization of the medical technology raises the possibility of useless and prolonged suffering during the last days, months, or even years.

Under these grim prospects, grassroots America seems to have few problems in affirming what seemed to be a logical extension of refusal and withdrawal, namely, curtailing the meaningless prolongation of life and suffering by means of physician-assisted suicide and/or voluntary euthanasia. Social institutions, on the other hand, have said, "Not so fast!" What appears to be a straightforward albeit tragic decision for the average American "on the street" is not so simple when the decision is cast as social policy. The three primary institutions constituting the social dynamics surrounding life and death have become embroiled in tremendous tensions about making decisions at the end of life. These institutions are:

1. Medicine, which maintains social understandings of good health;
2. Law, most responsible for maintaining good social order; and
3. Religion, which has functioned historically as the institution that watches over "good" dying.

All three of these institutions have complicated how individuals must handle decisionmaking in this country at the end of life. Any future improvements in our current malaise will depend on the interplay between these institutions.

Modern medicine has been quick to embrace, yet slow to adjust to, technological capabilities. Two of the most immediate problems have been resistance to do anything that shortens life and lack of attention to complaints about palliative care from patients or their families. Death is traditionally viewed as the Enemy to be conquered, with a capital "E." The idea of actively administering a treatment or refusing or withdrawing a treatment, the intentional result of which is death, is something antithetical to the motivations and drives of the medical establishment in this country. Families often complain about how easy it is to get their loved ones hooked up to sophisticated machinery, but that getting them disconnected takes an act of the state.[1] Change has come slowly and sometimes reluctantly. In what appears to be a first, the Oregon Medical Board disciplined a doctor for *under-treating* his patients' pain. The discipline imposed requires the doctor to complete a one-year program of having his practice assessed by another doctor, and a course on doctor-patient communications. The Chair of the Oregon Board of Medical Examiners, in commenting on the case, acknowledged that 20 years ago, the doctor would not have been brought before the board, but now there exists a new compassion regarding patients in pain (Associated Press, 1999). Despite the fanfare about informed consent and advance directives, evidence suggests that the last wishes of patients are still often overlooked. Advance directives are lost, ignored, or, because of some inadequacy in the form, are not honored (Knox, 1998). Secondly, despite calls to improve palliative care and many advances in medication measurement and management, the battle has been uphill (Coyle, 1990). A 1997 SUPPORT study of ICU patients indicates that 60% of their families reported that the patient experienced severe pain during the last three days of life (Lynn et al., 1997; SUPPORT, 1995). Between 10% and 50% of patients in programs *devoted to palliative care* still report significant pain one week before death (Quill, 1997). Common sense suggests that where no devoted program exists, the percentages are much higher.

Added to this is the neglected reality of psychological pain patients suffer when they continue living in spite of their wishes. Marshall Klavan (ironically, a physician) is suing a hospital where physicians ignored his instructions in a living will not to be kept alive on life support. In response to his attempted suicide, doctors resuscitated Klavan. A week later, he was taken off life support in accordance with his living will. When his condition worsened, physicians reversed their course by reconnecting him to life support. Klavan subsequently suffered a stroke. With a prognosis of a life expectancy of 18 more years, Klavan now lives totally dependent on others, not only in physical pain, but with the mental anguish of possibly living in a condition he explicitly tried to avoid (Associated Press, 1999).

A huge gulf exists between attitudes of institutional medicine and patients regarding the appropriateness of saving or prolonging life just because it is possible and what is perceived to be a lack of enough attention to pain and suffering at the end of life. Further, who should have the authority to make these ultimate decisions? To answer this question, American society has turned to the law. But our legal institutions have struggled to find any consistent or common approach to alleviating our ethical malaise.

From the beginning, it seems the courts were reluctant to step into these issues. As arbitrator of disputes, courts naturally focused on the issues in terms of "rights." The *Quinlan* decision contains specific expression of the court's reluctance, stating, "We consider that a practice of applying to a court to confirm such decisions would generally be inappropriate" (*Quinlan,* 1976). More than a quarter of a century later, we are engulfed in a litigious milieu with regard to end-of-life decisionmaking. The *Quinlan* court's cautions that such decisions best remain in the counsel of family-physician-patient relationships has been largely ignored. Courts are routinely called upon to sanction any move, out of fear of liability or disagreement, between the involved parties. Even when the patient's wishes are clearly and cogently expressed, the destination for decisionmaking often becomes the courtroom. We may not assume that the concerns of the patient or family will be acknowledged or carry any special weight. One of the most recent examples is the case of Hugh Finn in Virginia. Governor James Gilmore III became personally involved in blocking Mrs. Finn's attempts to withdraw a feeding tube from her husband (Baker, 1999) (*Finn v. Annaburg Manor,* 1998).

Odd contradictions result in our present state of affairs. A time traveler from the 1960s would be shocked to find that under certain circumstances we have to go to court to ask permission to die! Also, even though a body of case law has been collected respecting the patient's wishes to consent to or withdraw treatment, or the family's wishes for mentally incapacitated relatives, these precedents only apply to a narrow range of medical conditions. A person who is severely brain damaged, unconscious, unaware of any aspect of existence, and unable to feel suffering will have little trouble having treatments stopped. A severely brain-damaged person, however, who is somewhat aware and capable of some degree of interaction and suffering, will find it harder to have treatment stopped. If this same person were not diagnosed as terminally ill and could live for years in this condition, the chance for stopping treatment likely lessens. We have seen recent examples of this scenario in Michigan and California, in the cases of Michael Martin and Robert Wendland, respectively. The Michigan Supreme Court and the California court both denied petitions from their families to discontinue treatment because the patients, although severely and irreversibly brain-damaged and unable ever to recover any semblance of function, were nevertheless slightly conscious and not in a vegetative state. Nor, in technical terms, are they terminal, since prospects for continued existence in this state are indefinite. Unfortunately, PVS has become a kind of benchmark for allowing a person to be withdrawn from medical treatment much as brain death was decades ago. The logic of this thinking leads sadly to the following dictum: *The longer and more you suffer, the longer you have to live and the less your wishes are respected* (Cranford, 1999).

As the primary social institution of death, religion has played an awkward role. Our legal system presumes to rest on the deeply established foundation of the traditions and principles of Judaism and Christianity. Precisely how and to what extent this is so is beyond the scope of this essay. Both of these religions view human life with sanctity. Unfortunately, some have taken this to mean that life is sacred in any form or condition, thus leading religiously based groups to "save" patients from those (often family) who are trying to "kill" them by withdrawing treatment. Religious zeal to defend "the sanctity of life" has played a major role in the way end-of-life decisions have been shaped. This has been especially important in the cases of *Quinlan, Brophy, Cruzan, Busalacchi,* and *"BABY K."*

Patricia Brophy complained of so-called pro-life forces who fought her out of a religious ideology, while they ignored that she struggled to reach her decision to "let her husband go" in the context of her religious faith. She said: "Paul was not dead, but no longer alive either. They [pro-life groups] wanted me to force him to live. What moral obligation did Paul have to live like this?"[2] The court determined that she had discharged her duties as her husband's guardian "with the highest degree of ethical and moral exaction." Her priest testified that she reached her decision to withdraw treatment out of compassion and love (*Brophy,* 1986).

In total contrast, the *"BABY K"* case demonstrates how religion is used in order to demand the extraordinary treatment from which Patricia Brophy sought her husband's relief. BABY K was born anencephalic;[3] her mother demanded that all-out aggressive measures be taken to keep the baby alive as long as possible. Notwithstanding the fact that no medical treatment could ever improve BABY K's futile condition, the judgment by hospital physicians that such treatment was medically and ethically inappropriate, and the agreement of the father and BABY K's guardian ad litem with the physicians, the mother resisted any effort to refuse treatment. Why this intransigence? It was because of her religious stance. Court testimony sums up her position: "[The mother] has a firm Christian faith that all life should be protected. She believes that God will work a miracle if that is his will. Otherwise, [she] believes, God, and not other humans, should decide the moment of her daughter's death" (*In the Matter of BABY K.,* 1993). The U. S. Fourth Circuit Appeals Court ruled that the physicians must treat *BABY K, even though they considered it medically and ethically inappropriate* (!) (*In the Matter of BABY K.,* 1994).

These examples show the ambiguity that results in ethical judgment-making because of religion. Patricia Brophy's decisions were driven by the religious orientations of her husband and herself. At the same time, her most vociferous opposition would come from groups primarily motivated by *their* religious convictions. Taking a position opposite to that of Brophy, the mother of BABY K argued that her deep religious conviction was the moral basis for keeping her infant alive. Religion has not functioned to bring resolution to end-of-life cases, but has resulted in antagonism. The result so far is polarization, not solution.

TRAJECTORIES FOR CHANGE

Where do we go from here? Can a social consensus be reached for the best approach to such grave situations? Probably not. But some basic changes could improve the current state of morass. Medicine must find ways to transcend the defensive posture that has developed. A first step toward alleviating this defensiveness must be to re-examine the concept of death. The definition of death is biological. Might not medical science consider establishment of new standards for conceiving of patients in PVS and "minimally conscious states" as dead? Some within medicine, searching for a designation, refer to such patients as "non-dead, non-people." A thorough reassessment of models and definitions of death needs revisiting. Partial brain death and an asymptotic model have already begun some debate. It is fairly well known that the current model is primarily designed to facilitate procurement of transplantable organs, not to meet the needs of patients and their families as death approaches. The medical establishment must lead the way in providing a more holistic and meaningful approach than our current concept of death provides (Truog, 1997; Veatch, 1993).

Medicine needs to come to some realistic policy concerning futility. Currently, the concept revolves around probabilities and numbers. This creates the false impression that stopping treatment is about calculating the odds of whether it will work. But given existing abilities, decisions to treat or withdraw treatment are not about numbers but values. Virtually all decisions involve the weighing of a treatment's benefits against its burdens. Physicians should not pretend that the concept of futility is simply physiological. For families, this approach drives them to think in terms of "defying the odds." This steers the decisionmaking process the wrong way, away from doctor-patient discussions about real value decisions: patient wishes, burden versus benefits of treatment, encumbrance of resources, the true goals and expectations of medicine, and transparent discussions about social justice (Rubin, 1998). As Dr. Fred Plum, one of the formative researchers of PVS, stated, "We must some day face the brutal truth that the perpetual, demanded treatment of PVS patients is useless. It steals from the mouths of others who might have some hope."[4] Surely, medicine must be willing to act to uphold professional standards that guard the physician from becoming a technician, providing futile treatment on demand, or more likely, out of fear.

The courts are ill equipped to deal with end-of-life cases. As a general rule, no person at the end-of-life should have to seek a judge's permission to die. Stories of long, protracted court battles as well as a noticeable reticence among hospitals to give final decisionmaking power to families has resulted in a growing American sentiment that shouts: "Keep your laws off my body!" (GLS Research, 1998). What could the courts do to make this the extraordinary exception, instead of the all too common routine? The "clear and convincing evidence" standard adapted by the state supreme courts in New York, Missouri, Kentucky, and Michigan (and found to be constitutional by the U.S. Supreme Court in the Cruzan decision) is unrealistic and unworkable. It puts families far too much to the defensive, having to prove to the court why they *are not unworthy* of trust. The burden should be shifted onto the shoulders of those who would show a family or guardian is not acting in a trustworthy way regarding the patient. Trust should be assumed unless it can be shown otherwise. Gladly, in the cases *Guardianship of Doe* (1992) and *Fiori* (1996), a "substituted judgment standard" was used. This approach places basic trust in the family as most knowledgeable about the patient's preferences, goals, and values. When situations arise where no substituted judgment may be effectuated, a "standard of best interests" needs to be employed (*Fiori,* 1996). This primary shift would reduce litigation drastically. Our social institutions must find ways to include families as trusted members of tragic decisionmaking rather than treat their actions with suspicion.

What is religion's proper social role in end-of-life decisions? As we have seen, people appeal to religious beliefs to help them both justify ending treatment and to continue it in the most extreme conditions. In our opinion, religious institutions have so far "copped out" of making the kind of contributions they should make to social policies. Historically, Christianity led the way in providing society with revolutionary models of compassionate care for the dying and their families. At the end of the millennium, this has not been the case. Instead of building hospitals, major emphasis is directed to building large complexes to house mega-congregations. Business models for growing larger churches dominate. Health care has been supplanted by church growth.

A primary example of this change in emphasis is Hospice. When one visits a full service Hospice, all the circumstances presuppose religion. One might expect to be entering a religious setting. The focus is on helping people deal with dying head on, with compassion and patient/family involvement. Yet, to people from mainstream religious faiths, the atmosphere is almost surreal, because of the lack of religious orientation. A chapel attempts a universal appeal, with a minimum of symbols which are, as much as possible, neutral. By and large, Hospices are owned and operated as an arm of a hospital.

In truth, Hospice has filled a vacuum traditionally filled by religion. Hospices struggle, however, to gather funds to build a few units. Why have religious institutions abandoned any full fledged ministry in a society where end-of-life decisions have become paramount? Especially given our aging population, this lack of aggressive commitment seems indefensible.

The lack of institutional attention by some religious institutions has led to lack of theological depth or dialogue among them. Many of the demands made from religious conviction are ill-informed and show a lack of theological education. From a theological perspective, the demands made by BABY K's mother are not in the mainstream of Christian thinking. Such preservation of life trivializes the concept of personhood, the meaning of life, and thwarts social responsibility for others who may have benefitted by the medical resources they were denied. It also trivializes the integrity of those who must care for the dying. Nowhere within the historic streams of Christian theology do we have a duty to live or force others to live at all costs. Rather, a more central question has always been, "For what are you willing to die?" Christianity has a long tradition of understanding our individual autonomy in the context of the larger community. Religious institutions need to redirect their energies to learning how to educate, mediate, and communicate, instead of indoctrinate. Reverend Harry Cole exposes the emptiness of our current litigious approach, and the impact mature theological perspectives can make. He speaks about his own wife Jackie, who survived a massive intra cerebral hemorrhage:

> The premise that because Jackie was not clinically dead she was clinically alive, and as such should be treated as if a real purposeful life was at all possible, was one I could no longer accept. Nor could I accept the precise legal definition of life on which that premise was arguably based–a life measured by the results of two electroencephalograms, a life without regard for love or compassion or for what a fitting response would be when life was threatened with prolonged and unredemptive suffering. (Cole, 1988)

Religion already contains the framework for a less litigious social climate for end-of-life decisions. Its best orientations provide a healthy context for developing a meaningful and socially responsible understanding of substituted judgment, holistic concepts of personhood, and more adequate approaches to dealing with dying and death. Its major challenge is to reclaim these essential impulses.

America is currently struggling with how we as members of society die. We want to live long, but we want quality of life and a "good" death. Most issues circulate around tensions between the ability to extend life (quantity) and the meaningfulness that such an extended life may or may not have (quality). The challenges of decisionmaking have resulted in what is often conflicting values among medicine, law, and religion. We have suggested that each of these institutions must revisit some of its fundamental values if a more meaningful and satisfying social climate is to be created around end-of-life situations.

Medicine must be willing to function beyond calculating odds or practicing defensively, motivated by fear. The courts must recapture their earlier reluctance about becoming an agency granting permission for people to die (Quinlan). Absent evidence to the contrary, families should be empowered as trustworthy to carry out wishes of those who cannot speak for themselves, except in rare situations. Each religion must educate its adherents about the nature and place of death within its particular religious heritage. Less litigious or clinical approaches to dying are indigenous to religious traditions, tying the way we die to the purposes of life, personhood, and the larger social community. All three of these basic institutions of dying must recapture their historic social functions if dying in the new millennium is to become any more humane than it is now.

NOTES

1. Pete Busalacchi was forced to fight a long and expensive battle with the Supreme Court of Missouri in order to remove life support from his daughter, Christine; his charge is a good example. He comments on the discrepancy between getting treatment and removing treatment: "I did what any dad would do for their kid. I never had to ask the State what I could or should do. No permission was needed from any authority to hook my daughter up to feeding tubes, insert a tube in her brain, and a thousand other things." Quoted from personal statements made at a conference, "Managing Mortality," December 3-5, 1992, Center for Bioethics, University of Minnesota, Minneapolis.

2. Personal statement made by Mrs. Brophy, expressing her dismay toward people who wanted to enforce a legalistic view of life and death on her husband, and her power to interpret his wishes. "Managing Mortality," December 3-5, 1992.

3. Anencephaly is a congenital malformation in which a major portion of the brain, skull, and scalp are missing. The brain stem supports autonomic functions and reflex actions, but the lack of a cerebrum means BABY K is permanently unconscious.

4. Personal notes from conference on "Managing Mortality," 1992.

AUTHOR NOTES

D. Dixon Sutherland is Professor of Religious Studies and Director of the Institute for Christian Ethics at Stetson University. His research and writing spans early Christian history, philosophical theology, and ethics. His work seeks to understand mutual challenges between a relevant religious ethic and our contemporary society.

Rebecca C. Morgan is Professor of Law at Stetson University College of Law and Director of the Center for Law and Aging. She is also the immediate Past-President of the National Academy of Elder Law Attorneys and the co-author of Matthew Bender's *Tax, Estate, and Financial Planning for the Elderly* and the companion forms book. She has authored several articles on termination of treatment issues.

REFERENCES

A conference on managing mortality. (1992). Center for Bioethics, University of Minnesota, Minneapolis, December 3-5.

Associated Press. (1999, August 21). Doctor sues hospital for saving him.

In the Matter of BABY K., 832 F. Supp.1022 (Virginia, 1993).

In the Matter of BABY K., 16 F.3d 590 (Virginia, 1994).

Baker, D. (1999, January 28). Woman blasts officials' efforts to stop removal of feeding tube. *Washington Post*, B09.

Brophy v. New England Sinai Hospital, 497 N.E.2d 626, 632 (Mass. 1986).

Cole, H. (1988). Deciding on a time to die: A fitting response. *Second Opinion*, 7, 23.

Coyle, N., Adelhardt, J., Foley, K.M., Portenoy, R.K. (1990). Character of terminal illness in the advanced cancer patient: Pain and other symptoms during the last four weeks of life. *Journal of Pain and Symptom Management*, 5(2), 83-93.

Cranford, R. (1999). The more you suffer, the longer you live. *Bioethics Examiner*, 2(4), 1-2.

Finn v. Annaburg Manor, Nos. 39811, 44386, 44574 (1998).

GLS Research. (July, 1998). San Francisco. Full text available at <http://compassion indying.org/releases/survey.html>

Guardianship of Doe, 583 N.E.2d 1263 (Mass.1992).

In re Daniel Joseph Fiori, 543 Pa. 592, 673 A.2d 905 (Penn. 1996).

Knox, R. (1998, April 17). Patients' last wishes found often overlooked. *Boston Globe*, A01.

Lynn, J., Teno, J., Phillips, R., Wu, A., Desbiens, N., Harrold, J., Claessens, M., Wenger, N., Kreling, B., & Connors, A. (1997). Perceptions by family members of the dying experience of older and seriously ill patients. *Annals of Internal Medicine*, 126, 97-106.

Quinlan v. New Jersey, 355 A.2d 647 (N. J. 1976).

The SUPPORT Principal Investigators. A controlled trial to improve care for seriously ill hospitalized patients. The study to understand prognoses and preferences for outcomes and risks of treatments (SUPPORT). *Journal of the American Medical Association*, 274, 1591-1598.

Truog, R. (1997). Is it time to abandon brain death? *Hastings Center Report*, 27(1), 29-37.

Veatch, R. (1993). The impending collapse of the whole-brain definition of death. *Hastings Center Report*, 23(4), 18-24.

Wendland v. Supreme Court, 49 Cal. App. 4th 44 (Ct. App. 1996).

ECONOMIC SECURITY

The Continuing Gender Gap
in Later Life Economic Security

Leslie A. Morgan, PhD

University of Maryland Baltimore County

KEYWORDS. Poverty, elderly poor, economic insecurity, women and Social Security

Economic disadvantage and poverty among women in later life is not a new policy challenge in the United States (Burkhauser & Holden, 1982; Minkler & Stone, 1985). Higher rates of poverty, limited access to private pensions, and greater reliance on need-based transfer programs have been documented for the female majority of elders over many years and persist

Leslie A. Morgan is Professor and Chair, Department of Sociology and Anthropology, University of Maryland Baltimore County. Dr. Morgan's research focuses on later life families, marital transitions, gender, and housing alternatives for frail elders.

She can be contacted care of the Department of Sociology and Anthropology, University of Maryland Baltimore County, 345ACIV-B, 1000 Hilltop Circle, Baltimore, MD 21250 (E-mail: lmorgan@umbc.edu).

[Haworth co-indexing entry note]: "The Continuing Gender Gap in Later Life Economic Security." Morgan, Leslie A. Co-published simultaneously in *Journal of Aging & Social Policy* (The Haworth Press, Inc.) Vol. 11, No. 2/3, 2000, pp. 157-165; and: *Advancing Aging Policy as the 21st Century Begins* (ed: Francis G. Caro, Robert Morris, and Jill R. Norton) The Haworth Press, Inc., 2000, pp. 157-165. Single or multiple copies of this article are available for a fee from The Haworth Document Delivery Service [1-800-342-9678, 9:00 a.m. - 5:00 p.m. (EST). E-mail address: getinfo@haworthpressinc.com].

today, despite significant social changes. Data for 1997 showed that 7.0% of men 65 and older were at or below the poverty level, compared to 13.1% of women 65 and older and 22.4% of older women living alone (Dalaker & Naifeh, 1998). Unmarried women 65 and older rely on Social Security for 51% of their total income, compared to 39% for unmarried older men and 36% for older couples (Social Security Administration, 1998). For 25% of unmarried women in later life, Social Security is their only source of income (Social Security Administration, 1998). Women constitute about three quarters of the elderly who are recipients of SSI benefits (Social Security Administration, 1995). The risks of economic insecurity are not evenly divided among women, but are greatest for the oldest cohorts, those who are unmarried or with limited education (Dalaker & Naifeh, 1998; Shaw & Yi, 1997). Older African- and Hispanic-American women are, like their younger counterparts, at significantly higher risk of poverty (Choudhury & Leonesio, 1997).

Cross-national research suggests that a substantial gender differential is not inevitable in economically developed nations, but relates to the structure of U.S. income maintenance policies (Burkhauser & Smeeding, 1994). European countries provide a number of initiatives, including basic pensions, child-rearing credits, earnings sharing, and protections for the divorced that augment earnings-based benefits for women (Stapf, 1997). Nonetheless, equity remains a concern in developing and developed nations, and older women constitute a majority of the elderly poor in many countries worldwide that peg later-life income to earnings in the paid economy (Midgley, 1996; Stapf, 1997).

Understanding later-life economic disadvantage among women requires a life-course perspective (Choudhury & Leonesio, 1997). Women who fall into poverty in later life following major transition events, such as widowhood or major health problems, were most often poor at some stage in their earlier lives; it is their personal histories that leave them vulnerable to poverty in old age more than simply age-related transitions (Choudhury & Leonesio, 1997).

If the U.S. gap rested simply on policies and programs that discriminated based on gender, then resolutions would be at hand. Instead, the underpinning assumptions for later-life income supports are structured largely based on earnings in the labor force and years worked. This prompts us to focus attention on differential behaviors of women and men (often described as "choices") throughout life which, interacting with provisions of social policies, result in economic disadvantage to women in later life.

THE PROBLEM

Since the bulk of retirement income derives either directly or indirectly from employment, gender differences in employment opportunities and experience are key to understanding the greater economic vulnerability among older women. Data from the 1960s onward show a clear trend toward greater labor-force participation among women in most age groups except those 65 to 69, but differences remain. For example, half of women 55 to 64 (50.9%) were employed in 1997 compared to two thirds of men (67.6%) (Quinn, 1999). The major explanation for the labor-force difference between the sexes continues to derive from marital status and family responsibilities for women (Ruhm, 1990). Data on women aged 55 showed a clear, negative association between years of labor-force experience and number of children, although causation remains problematic (Feuerbach & Erdwins, 1994). Similarly data for caregiving to older kin suggest that women remain more likely to interrupt employment to serve as caregivers, an economically rational decision in the short-term, given their lower earnings (Kingson & O'Grady-LeShane, 1993; Sandell & Iams, 1994). Seldom are such decisions made with an eye to long-term retirement income (Kingson & O'Grady-LeShane, 1993). Interruptions reduce income and associated asset development, as well as create zero earning years in a Social Security earnings profile, to reduce a worker's benefit (Harrington Meyer, 1996). They also may short-circuit vesting, or job tenure required to maximize pension benefits (Johnson, Sambamoorthi, & Crystal, 1999).

Rising labor-force participation among younger cohorts of women has significantly increased those who are dually entitled to Social Security benefits as spouse or worker (Harrington Meyer, 1996), with most dually entitled women still selecting the larger spousal benefit. The premise of the traditional, single-earner household means that there is no premium paid for the family's second earner, and sometimes a penalty is exacted in terms of lower benefits (Weaver, 1997). The inequity of having two-earner couples subsidizing benefits for couples choosing a more traditional single-earner lifestyle has remained politically intractable to date.

Of growing importance are issues relating to economic security of divorced older women as cohorts where divorce is more prevalent enter later life. Divorced spouses, who have been a policy concern for decades, remain among the most economically disadvantaged groups receiving Social Security benefits (Weaver, 1997). Most older divorced women do not receive alimony and rely heavily on Social Security benefits (Crown, Mutschler, Schulz, & Loew, 1993). Social Security differentiates between widowed and divorced women in terms of benefits (66% of the benefit amount versus 50% for the divorced) (Weaver, 1997).

Routes to poverty for the divorced may differ from those for widows. Marriages may not last long enough to earn spousal benefits from Social Security or rights to pension. Asset accumulation may be hampered among divorced women with custody of children by nonpayment or incomplete payment of child support in early and mid-life. Gaps also remain in certain pensions programs that may mean limited or no benefits for divorced women despite a lengthy marriage (AARP, 1993). Payments from pensions at divorce may not be helpful to long-term economic security if, as sometimes occurs, they come as lump sums (AARP, 1993). Although most states recognize a pension as a major marital asset to be allocated in the property settlement, the recency of most states' provisions means that many couples had divorced before such provisions became common (AARP, 1993).

PROPOSED CHANGES

We can look to no "silver bullet" to remedy a situation with complex roots in policies built on sometimes-outdated notions regarding gender and family. The major changes in family roles and labor-force behaviors are unlikely to generate equity in the near term without policy changes. Women continue to pursue life cycle choices (with encouragement of the gender gaps in wages and employment and the expectations of family and gender) that are inconsistent with a system of retirement income security based on labor-force participation. There is little short-term hope that these risks will be shared equitably by the sexes. Instead, there are proposed changes in existing policies likely to marginally improve the situation or to target especially disadvantaged groups. They follow, organized on the three major sources of later-life income: Social Security, private pensions, and earnings.

Social Security

Proposals either to share earnings between spouses or to increase the number of dropout years have been discussed for many years as remedies to problems of equity by analysts and policymakers (Congressional Budget Office, 1986; Sandell & Iams, 1994). Earnings sharing is argued by many to be the most efficient means of accommodating women's varied roles in the family and the labor force during marriage and making a move toward more adequate benefits in the case of divorce. Dollars earned by the couple are divided and credited toward individuals' Social Security benefits, regardless of who earned them (Congressional Budget Office, 1986).

Other proposals target particular groups. One budget-neutral proposal (Burkhauser & Smeeding, 1994; Sandell & Iams, 1997), increases Social Security benefits to survivors (primarily women) through an offsetting, modest decrease in the couple's benefits prior to widowhood. Burkhauser and Smeeding suggest that survivors receive a benefit equal to 75% (as opposed to the current 66%) of the joint benefit and simply shift benefit dollars toward the survivor (1994). Various forms of this proposal have been developed, but have faced political opposition in Congress (Burkhauser & Smeeding, 1994; Sandell & Iams, 1997). A similar proposal to increase benefits for divorced women to 75% of the ex-spouse's benefit would target the poorest of older women, but has no clear cost-neutral trade-off for its financing (Weaver, 1997).

Proposals to revise Social Security to include elements of privatization have been critiqued on the grounds that some would increase risks to women by lengthening the years of employment basis for Social Security from 35 to 38 and by providing fewer guarantees with regard to either risks connected with lump-sum payouts or couples' sharing of individually controlled retirement savings accounts (Rix & Williamson, 1998). The potentials to alter the redistributive effects of Social Security would also increase risks to Social Security benefits for women (Choudhury & Leonesio, 1997; Rix & Williamson, 1998). Advocates have begun to represent special concerns of women in these issues, but it is unclear whether provisions will be included to address gender-related concerns.

Pensions

Changes in private pensions, already under way, are likely to be driven by market forces rather than concerns over gender equity. Innovations, such as easing penalties in defined-benefit pension programs for those taking family leave as caregivers, are likely only to be enacted by employers attempting to keep skilled workers' loyalty in a highly competitive market (Korczyk, 1993). The move to defined-contribution pensions requires an understanding of markets and investing less common among women and working class and minority individuals. Barring better education, these groups could face higher risks in the move to employee-managed defined-contribution pensions (Rix & Williamson, 1998). In addition, purchase of annuities with lump sums from defined-contribution plans may result in lower benefit amounts, due to women's greater longevity (Rix & Williamson, 1998).

Pension wealth continues to be significantly higher for male than female workers in the pre-retirement years (Johnson et al., 1999). Most of the ongoing gap in pension coverage can be attributed to the gender gap in wages and its correlation with pension availability across industries and sectors of the economy (Johnson et al., 1999). Ironically, we are moving toward more equity in pension coverage, because it is declining for men, not because it is improving for women (Reno, 1993). This suggests that both women and men will need to take action to replace this critical component of retirement income in future cohorts. Greater flexibility for individual retirement accounts will benefit only those with sufficient disposable income to save, again disadvantaging women.

Earnings

Wages constitute a significant portion of income for those beyond age 65, especially those in the upper ranges of income (Social Security Administration, 1994). Opportunities for employment beyond 65 for women both able and interested in such opportunities are likely to be increasingly viable (in human capital terms) in the future. Some major barriers to employment after retirement have already been lifted, with an increase in the Social Security earnings test amount from $13,500 in 1997 to $30,000 by 2002 for workers ages 65 to 69 and increases in the delayed retirement credit. In addition, the shift toward defined-contribution pension programs means that fewer pensions will contain financial disincentives for working past age 65 (Burkhauser & Quinn, 1997).

These changes may not effectively resolve problems for women, however, if discrimination in employment based on age, disability, or gender results in only poorly paid or undesirable employment options. To be useful to the most economically vulnerable women, labor-force opportunities must be protected with adequate funding for enforcement against these forms of discrimination. Continued attention to a safety net, beyond income maintenance provisions that are based on employment, remains especially important to women.

DISCUSSION

Social policies face barriers in redressing gender inequities in later-life economic well-being. Certain issues, such as the longevity of women, with its risk of outliving financial resources, are not amenable to easy solutions. Fundamental problems, such as a lifetime of lower wages, remain problematic in wage-based systems, especially for women spending most of their adult lives unmarried (Harrington Meyer, 1996). Differential rates of physical disability for women also limit the use of earnings-based systems to resolve inequity (Crimmins, Reynolds, & Saito, 1999).

Our income support system for older adults is based on employment history and earnings. These employment-based policies serve as the fulcrum for tipping the balance between economic security and insecurity. Unless employers, policymakers and the rest of us envision older workers as including a large percentage of women, we risk serious errors that could perpetuate the economic disadvantages for the female majority of older adults.

Politicians remain fixed on protecting diverse choices for women, ranging from pursuit of traditional homemaking to full-time career involvement, yet continue a system in which income maintenance remains predicated on paid employment. Dropout years are declining, but the problems of the wage, pension coverage, and hours-worked gaps are resistant to change. The protections of marriage can no longer be relied upon as the safety net for women, nor can we assume that employment equity is just around the corner.

To promote economic gender equity, I propose that revisions to the Social Security system include:

- An earnings-sharing system, which would shift benefits from an "earning/dependent spouse" viewpoint to a reflection of earnings as truly shared by the couple during marriage;
- Shifting dollars from couples to widows through alteration in the calculation of benefits to guarantee widows 75% of the couple benefit as previously described;
- Identifying funds to increase the benefit for a divorced spouse from 50% to 75% (equal to a widow's benefit) for qualifying marriages; and
- Conducting research in advance on the consequences for women, minorities, and other specific groups of changes, such as privatization.

In terms of pensions, it would be important to:

- Provide public education with regard to the importance of a pension as a portion of the divorce settlement for women;
- Develop policies to encourage the expansion of employer-sponsored pensions to expand coverage, which would benefit both sexes; and
- Encourage public education about investing targeted toward women.

To enhance the potential for earnings, key steps include:

- Ensuring sufficient funding to the EEOC for enforcement of age and sex discrimination laws; and
- Educating employers as to the positive successful models for retaining employees beyond traditional retirement ages.

Certain proposals, such as using SSI or a minimum Social Security benefit to address these problems, are probably not acceptable politically, given the negative views of needs-based programs (Sandell & Iams, 1997). Changes such as earnings sharing under Social Security or improving divorced or widow benefits are likely to bring about the quickest and most effective change (Sandell & Iams, 1994). Given the political climate, wherein discussions of restructuring and financing of major programs such as Social Security and Medicare take up most of the energy, issues of equity by gender often fall by the wayside. Initiatives to address gaps, inconsistencies and "structural lag" in several of these programs are required to insure that the coming cohorts of women approach the systems for later-life income maintenance with a more even playing field.

REFERENCES

American Association of Retired Persons, Women's Initiative. (1993). *Women, pensions & divorce: Small reforms that could make a big difference.* Washington, DC: Author.

Burkhauser, R.V., & Holden, K.C. (Eds.) (1982). *A challenge to Social Security: The changing roles of women and men in American society.* New York: Academic Press.

Burkhauser, R.V., & Quinn, J.F. (1997). *Pro-work policy proposals for older Americans in the 21st century.* Policy Brief No 9/1997. Syracuse, NY: Syracuse University Center for Policy Research.

Burkhauser, R.V., & Smeeding, T.M. (1994). *Social Security reform: A budget neutral approach to reducing older women's disproportionate risk of poverty.* Policy Brief No 2/1994, Syracuse, NY: Syracuse University Center for Policy Research.

Choudhury, S., & Leonesio, M.V. (1997). Life cycle aspects of poverty among older women. *Social Security Bulletin,* 60 (2),17-36.

Congressional Budget Office, Congress of the United States. (1986). *Earnings sharing options for the Social Security system.* Washington, DC: USGPO.

Crimmins, E.M., Reynolds, S.L. & Saito, Y. (1999). Trends in health and ability to work among the older working-age population. *Journal of Gerontology: Social Sciences,* 54B (1), S31-40.

Crown, W.H., Mutschler, P.H., Schulz, J.H., & Loew, R. (1993). *The economic status of divorced older women.* Waltham, MA: Heller School, Brandeis University.

Dalaker, J., & Naifeh, M. (1998). *Poverty in the United States: 1997.* U.S. Bureau of the Census, Current Population Reports, Series P60-201. Washington, DC: USGPO.

Feuerbach, E.J., &. Erdwins, C.J. (1994). Women's retirement: The influence of work history. *Journal of Women and Aging,* 6(3), 69-85.

Harrington Meyer, M. (1996). Making claims as workers or wives: The distribution of Social Security benefits. *American Sociological Review,* 61, 449-465.

Johnson, R.W., Sambamoorthi, U., & Crystal S. (1999). Gender differences in pension wealth: Estimates using provider data. *The Gerontologist,* 39(3), 320-333.

Kingson, E.R., & O'Grady-LeShane, R. (1993). The effects of caregiving on women's Social Security benefits. *The Gerontologist,* 33 (2), 230-239.

Korczyk, S.M. (1993). Gender issues in employer pensions policy. In R.V. Burkhauser and D.L. Salisbury (Eds.), *Pensions in a changing economy* (pp. 59-65). Washington, DC: Employee Benefit Research Institute.

Midgely, J. (1996). Challenges facing Social Security. In J. Midgely and M.B. Tracy (Eds.), *Challenges to Social Security: An international exploration* (pp. 1-18). Westport, CT: Auburn House.

Minkler, M., & Stone, R. (1985). The feminization of poverty and older women. *The Gerontologist,* 25 (4), 351-357.

Quinn, J. (1999). *Retirement patterns and bridge jobs in the 1990s.* Washington, DC: Employee Benefit Research Benefit Institute.

Reno, V.P. (1993). The role of pensions in retirement income. In R.V. Burkhauser and D.L. Salisbury (Eds.), *Pensions in a changing economy* (pp. 19-32). Washington, DC: Employee Benefit Research Institute.

Rix, S.E., & Williamson, J.B. (1998). *Social Security reform: How might women fare?* Washington, DC: AARP Public Policy Institute.

Ruhm, C.J. (1990). Career jobs, bridge employment, and retirement. In P. B. Doeringer (Ed.), *Bridges to retirement: Older workers in a changing labor market* (pp. 92-107). Ithaca, NY: Cornell University/ILR Press.

Sandell, S.H., & Iams, H.M. (1994). Caregiving and women's Social Security benefits: A comment on Kingson and O'Grady-LeShane. *The Gerontologist, 34*(5), 680-684.

Sandell, S.H. & Iams, H.M. (1997). Reducing women's poverty by shifting Social Security Benefits from retired couples to widows. *Journal of Policy Analysis and Management, 16* (2), 279-297.

Shaw, L.B. & Yi, H. (1997). How elderly women become poor: Findings from the New Beneficiary Data System. *Social Security Bulletin,* 60 (4), 46-50.

Social Security Administration. (1994). *Annual statistical supplement, 1994.* Washington, DC: USGPO.

Social Security Administration. (1995). *Annual statistical supplement, 1995.* Washington, DC: USGPO.

Social Security Administration. (1998). *Women and retirement security/*Cited 8/23/99 from http://www.ssa.gov/policy/womenrs.html.

Stapf, H. (1997). Old age poverty in selected countries of the European Union–Are women disproportionally affected? In N. Ott and G.G. Wagner (Eds.), *Income inequality and poverty in eastern and western Europe.* Heidelberg: Physica-Verlag.

Weaver, D.A. (1997). The economic well-being of Social Security beneficiaries, with an emphasis on divorced beneficiaries. *Social Security Bulletin,* 60 (4), 3-17.

AGING PRISONERS

The Elderly and Prison Policy

Jeff Yates, JD, PhD
William Gillespie, MA

University of Georgia
Athens, Georgia

KEYWORDS. Prison populations, elderly prisoners, first offense, prison sentences, end-of-life care, POPS (Project for Older Prisoners)

A white-haired 72-year-old man negotiates his wheelchair down a ramp. He makes his way over to a line that has formed in the common room in front of the nurse who is dispensing medicine to other elderly men who are patiently waiting. Some of the men are in wheelchairs or use walkers, and some can

Jeff Yates is an attorney and Assistant Professor in the Political Science Department at the University of Georgia. He has published articles on judicial politics, criminal justice, and aging policy.

William Gillespie earned an MA at the University of Arkansas (1998) and is a graduate student in Political Science at the University of Georgia, where he specializes in American politics.

Jeff Yates can be contacted care of the Political Science Department, University of Georgia, Athens, GA 30602 (E-mail: jyates@arches.uga.edu).

[Haworth co-indexing entry note]: "The Elderly and Prison Policy." Yates, Jeff, and William Gillespie. Co-published simultaneously in *Journal of Aging & Social Policy* (The Haworth Press, Inc.) Vol. 11, No. 2/3, 2000, pp. 167-175; and: *Advancing Aging Policy as the 21st Century Begins* (ed: Francis G. Caro, Robert Morris, and Jill R. Norton) The Haworth Press, Inc., 2000, pp. 167-175. Single or multiple copies of this article are available for a fee from The Haworth Document Delivery Service [1-800-342-9678, 9:00 a.m. - 5:00 p.m. (EST). E-mail address: getinfo@haworthpressinc.com].

stand on their own, but all suffer from at least some of the infirmities commonly associated with old age. At the other end of the room, an elderly man suffering from Alzheimer's disease is calmed down after experiencing an anxiety attack. While this hypothetical scenario might reasonably lead one to conclude that the description is that of a nursing home, it could actually be an appropriate depiction of a scene from one of our nation's prisons, where the line between corrections and convalescent care has become blurred.[1]

America's prisons are experiencing a significant increase in the number of elderly prisoners that they deal with. This increase in "graying" prisoners brings with it a host of policy issues that must be dealt with, including cost containment, health care concerns, and justice considerations. In this article, we present this increase in the elderly prison population as a burgeoning policy concern. We also examine some of the means that have been used to deal with the problems posed by an aging prison population and offer some alternative solutions to dealing with this situation.

THE DILEMMA OF AGING PRISON POPULATIONS

As demonstrated in Figure 1, it is evident that the number of elderly prisoners has risen substantially in the 1980s and 1990s, and will likely continue to rise if projected estimates hold true. The upward trend in elderly prisoners shown in Figure 1 adjures the question of why we are finding more elderly people in our nation's prisons. To begin with, elderly prisoners typically fit one of two profiles. The first is the prisoner who has spent a substantial portion of his life in the prison system, either due to a long sentence for a serious crime or due to a pattern of recidivism for less serious crimes. These inmates have grown old in prison and have become "institutionalized," meaning that they have come to regard prison as home. The second is the prisoner who is incarcerated due to a "first-offense" crime committed late in life (e.g., Goetting, 1983). A growing literature details the problem of the cognitive disabilities of the elderly that may be associated with dementia, aggressiveness, and loss of inhibitions (e.g., Aday, 1994). These disabilities can result in ordinarily law-abiding elderly citizens committing crimes for the first time in their lives. Such prisoners have often committed serious crimes (e.g., assault, murder, sexual offenses, etc.) for which probation or intermediate sanctions are not presently viable sentencing options.

With these two types of elderly offenders in mind we can address the causes of the increase in elderly prison populations. Essentially, the bulk of the increase in elderly prisoners can be attributed to demographic changes and general criminal justice policy changes over time. First, the nation is experiencing a rise in the number of elderly citizens generally. It is estimated that there are currently more than 57 million citizens over the age of 55, and it

FIGURE 1. Current and Projected Total Inmates Over 55 Years Old from 1985-2010

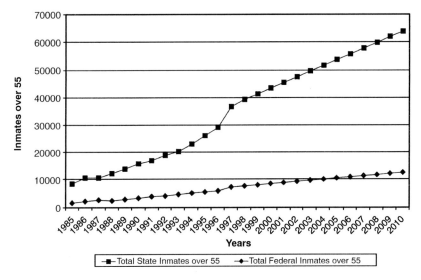

Source: American Correctional Association, 1999.

is projected that there will be more than 74 million people in this age group, comprising approximately 25% of the general population, by the year 2010 (U.S. Bureau of the Census, 1996). This demographic trend may be associated with increases in both of the types of elderly prisoners just discussed. Career prisoners of this growing demographic subgroup are now coming into their senior years within the confines of America's penitentiaries. Further, as the total number of seniors in the general population increases, it is reasonable to expect that there will be more senior first offenders for the criminal justice system to deal with as well.

Also at the root of the proliferation in elderly prisoners are increasingly harsh criminal justice policies that may have particularly deleterious consequences for elderly offenders. The efforts of political leaders and public fear of crime have led the federal government and the states to institute "get tough" policies for punishing offenders. The political movement that has led to these policies mirrors an underlying paradigmatic shift that has been going on in the criminal justice discipline since the 1970s, which sees rehabilitative corrections goals being replaced by the goals of retribution and incapacitation. These "get tough" policies include determinant sentencing, mandatory minimums and sentencing guidelines, and the recent "three strikes" laws for habitual offenders. While each of these policies has its own unique history and theoretical purpose, they are all essentially designed to restrict (or nullify) the discretion of criminal justice actors who are often perceived by the public and politicians as being too soft on offenders. Thus, such policies diminish the ability of judges and parole boards to take into account mitigating individual characteristics, such as old age, in computing the length of an offender's sentence.

While long prison sentences can serve the purpose of protecting the public from young offenders and perhaps deterring young offenders from future crime, their application to elderly offenders seems incongruous. The elderly are not likely to be offending again and a moderate to long sentence (e.g., 10-20 years) can effectively become a life sentence for someone in his senior years (Long, 1994). Elderly prisoners may even get an unfair deal in state criminal justice systems that use indeterminant (discretionary) sentencing. In such systems it is often the case that parole is, either explicitly or implicitly, conditioned on prisoners' voluntary involvement in a rehabilitation program such as higher education or vocational training courses. Of course, these programs have little practical benefit for prisoners either at or approaching retirement age. Hence, elderly prisoners often show little interest in rehabilitation programs and as a result may not fare well in parole decisions. Furthermore, another important consideration in parole decisions is the potential of the inmate to secure post-incarceration employment and housing. Of course, parole expectations concerning employment are higher for those inmates under the age of 60 than for those at or nearing retirement age. However, both age groups are likely to experience substantial barriers in the job and/or housing markets due to their two-fold disadvantage: They are old and they have a prison record. Since many elderly prisoners have few remaining ties to the outside world and face such barriers to employment and housing, their ability to gain parole may be jeopardized, and they may not even want it if it is offered (Goetting, 1983).

The costs of keeping the elderly in prison can be staggering. While the cost of keeping a young adult in prison, about $20,000 per year, seems high to many people, the cost of keeping an elderly person in prison typically runs over three times that amount (see Dubler, 1998; Ornduff, 1996). The specialized medical requirements of elderly prisoners vary from simple needs such as hearing aids and dentures to more expensive items such as high-cost prescription medication, prosthetic devices, and wheelchairs. At the far end of the cost spectrum are the needs of Alzheimer's sufferers and critically or terminally ill prisoners. While it might be rationalized that elderly health care is costly regardless of setting, it is important to note that the transactional costs to the public for providing such care in a prison setting (e.g., security, transportation, etc.) greatly compound the usual costs of treatment (Ornduff, 1996).

In order for correctional institutions to keep up with the minimum requirements of the Americans with Disabilities Act, prisons will likely experience increased costs in facility modifications to accommodate the needs of elderly disabled prisoners (see Adams, 1995). Further, the U.S. Supreme Court's decision in *Estelle v. Gamble* (1976) requires that prison officials provide for inmates' medical care under the Eighth Amendment's protections against cruel and unusual punishment. While *Estelle*'s legal requirement that prison officials not act in "deliberate indifference" to prisoners' medical needs may seem rather minimal, subsequent lower court cases suggest that the federal courts are ready and willing to require that correctional facilities take the necessary steps to ensure that inmates are provided with a healthy environment that accommodates their medical needs (Schmalleger, 1999, pp. 544-45). With the projected increase in geriatric prisoners, even the Supreme Court's rather minimal requirements in *Estelle* will necessitate significant increases in prisoner medical care outlays in the coming decades for correctional facilities to comport with the Eighth Amendment.

Beyond the monetary costs involved with incarcerating the elderly are the personal costs incurred by the elderly inmates. Studies of elderly prisoners report that they suffer from anxiety over the prospect of dying in prison as well as general feelings of depression and loneliness (e.g., Aday, 1994). Further, elderly inmates are sometimes preyed upon by more able-bodied young inmates and often have trouble keeping up with physically intensive work assignments that are more suited to younger inmates. Perhaps the most troublesome situation for elderly inmates involves the prospect of end-of-life care in prison. While society has generally experienced significant advances in palliative care and end-of-life treatment in recent decades, many such advances have not been extended to prisons. Prisoners approaching the end of their lives are often without adequate medical attention, legal planning counsel (e.g., advance directives, do-not-resuscitate orders, estate planning, etc.), and access to visitors (Dubler, 1998).

DEALING WITH THE PROBLEM

Coming to grips with the increase in aging prisoners in the United States means that state correctional agencies and other groups may need to explore policy alternatives in order to effectively deal with the increasing population of elderly prisoners. A number of states have dealt with the rising population of elderly inmates by creating separate facilities for them, thus segregating them from younger, perhaps more able-bodied, inmates (Adams, 1995; Goetting, 1995). The positives of segregating elderly inmates come from protecting vulnerable elderly inmates from more violent younger inmates, ease in offering specific programs for elderly inmates, and reduced emotional problems for elderly inmates. However, this approach is not without drawbacks. One reason that prison officials may be reluctant to segregate elderly inmates is that older inmates may serve a functional purpose in age-integrated systems in that they calm younger inmates and serve as positive role models. Furthermore, segregation may also mean that older inmates are excluded from prison work assignments and vocational training programs that some elderly inmates find fulfilling. Lastly, the implicit assumption underlying age segregation, that elderly inmates can be appropriately considered as a homogeneous group with substantially similar needs, may be inaccurate. While segregation may be very suitable for sick and frail elderly inmates, other senior inmates may have few problems in an integrated environment and may actually prefer having senior status among younger inmates. Still another distinction among elderly inmates can be found in the cultural and behavioral differences between those elderly inmates who have spent extensive time in prison versus those elderly inmates who have been only recently convicted of crimes. Gennaro Vito and Deborah Wilson (1985) note that elderly inmates are a heterogeneous group and suggest that a variety of approaches to handling such inmates may be necessary.

An innovative program addressing rising elderly prisoner populations is called **POPS** (the Project for Older Prisoners). Professor Jonathan Turley began **POPS** at Tulane University to seek the early release of inmates over the age of 55 who have already served the average sentence for their offense and are unlikely to repeat their crimes. This program seeks to guarantee that released prisoners do not commit new crimes through a stringent screening process and by ensuring that help is available for released clients for things such as finding jobs, housing, and access to Social Security payments (Ornduff, 1996). The POPS program operates as a voluntary organization, which relies upon chapters at law schools to provide law student volunteers who screen and evaluate appropriate candidates for early release. The POPS program's impact on state prison policy remains minor because many states do not have chapters, and the tight screening of inmates for release further limits potential amelioration of aging state prison populations. However, POPS does serve as a model for how state programs could be designed to promote the release of certain appropriate elderly inmates back into society. While inmate-release programs are somewhat controversial, programs specifically tailored for elderly inmates can give state correctional authorities some relief from prison overcrowding and soaring medical budgets. Federal and state funding of **POPS**-type release programs are needed to help implement programs like this in all states. Given the projected increase in elderly prisoners in coming years, such an investment would reap dividends by freeing up prison space to use for younger, more threatening offenders.

Prisons can also alleviate overcrowding and healthcare costs through specialized "medical parole" programs for elderly inmates. These paroles, sometimes called "compassionate release" by advocates, are granted to those prisoners who are terminally ill or require extensive medical care that cannot be adequately provided in a prison setting (Dubler, 1998). While these programs exist in most states, no constitutional right to parole for medical conditions has been recognized by the courts. Because medical paroles and releases are aimed at severely or terminally ill inmates, they are not particularly controversial. However, the limits on the potential recipients to medical parole and release make the benefits to prison overcrowding concerns and increased medical costs for elderly inmates minimal.

We believe that age-based sentencing reforms, or simply restoring judicial discretion in sentencing older inmates, seems to offer the most potential benefit to reducing (or at least slowing the increase) of elderly prison populations. Thomas Long (1994) describes the by-product of the Federal Sentencing Reform Act of 1984 as making age largely irrelevant as a factor to determining sentence length. Instead, the particular characteristics of the crime at issue become the factors that judges use for sentencing, rather than the offender characteristics. Long does note that §5H1.1 of the Federal Sentencing Guidelines indicates that age may be relevant in extraordinary cases, and that extraordinary cases are cases in which the offender is elderly and infirm and where punishment may be meted more efficiently and less costly by other means than incarceration (Long, 1994, p. 4). However, while these provisions technically give federal judges discretion in cases involving the elderly, in practice the "extraordinary" requirement has had a chilling effect on judicial discretion, and age has practically ceased to be a mitigating factor in sentencing since the guidelines were amended.

Returning discretion to federal judges, at least for consideration of age and health as a factor in sentencing elderly offenders, is warranted. Granting broader judicial discretion in this narrow area will increase the likelihood of shorter or alternative sentences for the elderly, thus relieving prisons of overcrowding and expensive elderly care. At the state level, some sentencing guidelines allow for age to serve as a mitigating factor; however, typically little guidance is provided as to when age is an appropriate consideration, hence the use of age as a factor in sentencing may vary widely depending upon the views of the trial judge involved (Long, 1994; Ornduff, 1994). Of course, some elderly offenders do pose a serious threat to society and hence are not appropriate candidates for lenient sentencing or early release. However, these elderly offenders tend to be the exception rather than the rule. The typical recidivism rate for prisoners 18-24 years of age is approximately

22%, whereas the recidivism rate for released prisoners over the age of 45 is only about 2% (Turley, 1989). Thus, the recent punitive trends in sentencing reform (mandatory minimums, three strikes, etc.) should be tempered with a presumption of leniency for offenders in their senior years. Judges could use their common sense and discretion to sort out situations in which the specific characteristics of the individual offender or crime suggest that the presumption of leniency would not be appropriate.

The use of age as a mitigating factor in sentencing can be controversial. Critics argue that age and wisdom presumably make older inmates more culpable than younger inmates. Advocates of elderly defendants argue that equal sentences for elderly and young offenders can be unfair in practical effect because older offenders have fewer years of life remaining and hence, such sentences are disproportionately harsh for the elderly. While sentencing reforms offer perhaps the best chance at a large-scale impact on reducing elderly inmate populations, this policy alternative may be particularly controversial in that it involves important normative judgments about the nature of punishment and appropriate goals of the criminal justice system.

In conclusion, society must weigh its need to keep elderly inmates behind bars against its need for other social programs. Limited government budgets mean tradeoffs, so that every dollar spent for prison building and incarceration services means fewer dollars available for education or developing our economic infrastructure. This being the case, the increased costs of medical care for elderly inmates and the impending costs for prison expansion and renovation in coming years may outweigh the benefits society receives from locking up the elderly. Some argue that to explore alternative sentences and release policies for elderly inmates means that the crime itself has been deemed less serious and the victim discounted. However, in an era in which prison overcrowding concerns often require corrections officials to release youthful violent offenders who are likely to cause serious harm to society upon release, it seems especially nonsensical to keep geriatric inmates behind bars for arbitrarily extended periods of time for the purpose of retribution. Ultimately, the question of whether to incarcerate increasing numbers of elderly offenders turns on the values that a society chooses to honor.

NOTE

1. This hypothetical scenario is based on the real-life observations of Tammerlin Drummond (1999) when he visited the geriatric wing of a prison near Pittsburgh, Pennsylvania. He notes that increased demand for beds has prompted officials to plan a $23 million expansion of the facility that will triple its capacity.

REFERENCES

Adams, Jr., W. E. (1995). The incarceration of older criminals: Balancing safety, cost and humanitarian concerns. *Nova Law Review, 19,* 465.

Aday, R. H. (1994). Aging in prison: A case study of new elderly offenders. *International Journal of Offender Therapy and Comparative Criminology, 38,* 79.

American Correctional Association. (1999). *Directory–Juvenile & Adult Correctional Departments, Institutions, Agencies & Paroling Authorities.* Laurel, MD: Author.

Drummond, T. (1999, June 21). Cellblock seniors: They have grown old and frail in prison. Must they still be locked up? *Time,* p. 60.

Dubler, N. N. (1998). The collision of confinement and care: End-of-life care in prisons and jails. *Journal of Law, Medicine, and Ethics, 26,* 149.

Goetting, A. (1983). The elderly in prison: Issues and perspectives. *Journal of Research in Crime and Delinquency, 20,* 291.

Long, T. A. (1994). The federal sentencing guidelines and elderly offenders: Walking a tightrope between uniformity and discretion (and slipping). *Elder Law Journal, 2,* 69.

Ornduff, J. S. (1996). Releasing the elderly inmate: A solution to prison overcrowding. *Elder Law Journal, 4,* 173.

Schmalleger, F. (1999). *Criminal justice today.* New Jersey: Prentice-Hall.

Turley, J. (1989, October 9). Prisons aren't nursing homes. *The New York Times,* p. 17.

U.S. Bureau of the Census. (1996). Population Projections of the United States by Age, Sex, Race, and Hispanic Origin 1995-2050. *P25-1130.* Washington, DC: US GPO.

Vito, G. & Wilson, D. (1985). Forgotten people: Elderly inmates. *Federal Probation, 49,* 18.

LATINO ELDERS

Policy Development and the Older Latino Population in the 21st Century

Jan E. Mutchler, PhD

University of Massachusetts Boston

Jacqueline L. Angel, PhD

University of Texas at Austin

KEYWORDS. Hispanics, Latinos, immigration, citizenship, informal caregiving

---

Jan E. Mutchler is Associate Professor in Gerontology at the University of Massachusetts and a Fellow in its Gerontology Institute.

Jacqueline L. Angel is Assistant Professor at the Lyndon B. Johnson School of Public Affairs at the University of Texas at Austin.

Jan E. Mutchler can be contacted care of the Gerontology Institute, University of Massachusetts Boston, 100 Morrissey Boulevard, Boston, MA 02125-3393 (E-mail: jan.mutchler@umb.edu).

[Haworth co-indexing entry note]: "Policy Development and the Older Latino Population in the 21st Century." Mutchler, Jan E., and Jacqueline L. Angel. Co-published simultaneously in *Journal of Aging & Social Policy* (The Haworth Press, Inc.) Vol. 11, No. 2/3, 2000, pp. 177-188; and: *Advancing Aging Policy as the 21st Century Begins* (ed: Francis G. Caro, Robert Morris, and Jill R. Norton) The Haworth Press, Inc., 2000, pp. 177-188. Single or multiple copies of this article are available for a fee from The Haworth Document Delivery Service [1-800-342-9678, 9:00 a.m. - 5:00 p.m. (EST). E-mail address: getinfo@haworthpressinc.com].

The growing diversity of the older population has considerable significance for policy development and planning. In this commentary, we develop three themes especially relevant to the older Latino population in the United States. First, we discuss the characteristics of this population most relevant for policy and planning. Among these characteristics are those relating to age structure, immigration and citizenship, socioeconomic status, and language use. Discussed next are the major programs supporting the health and economic well-being of the older population as they relate to older Latinos. Insofar as the access of Latinos to these programs has been limited, negative consequences for the population's well-being have resulted. Finally, we offer some observations, goals, and recommendations relating to the older Latino population as it evolves over the next decade.

While our discussion is cast in terms of the Latino population, we note that the themes we develop have broader national relevance. For example, the issues we cite associated with immigration and citizenship are relevant to other groups with sizable noncitizen components, such as the Asian population. Similarly, issues revolving around access to means-tested programs are of concern not only to lower-income Latinos and their families, but also to economically marginal elders of all ethnic backgrounds in the United States. Yet due to its size and anticipated growth, the Latino population–including individuals of Mexican, Puerto Rican, Cuban, and other Spanish descent–is a segment of the older population requiring special attention. Taken as a whole, the Latino population 65 and over is expected to increase from 1.5 million in 1995 to almost 14 million by 2050. By the year 2030, Latinos over the age of 65 will surpass African-Americans as the nation's largest group of older minorities (Siegel, 1999).

A PROFILE OF THE OLDER LATINO POPULATION

Several key aspects of this population are relevant to the development of policy in the coming years. One characteristic critical for gerontologists to understand is the relative youth of the Latino population in the United States. The median age of Latinos in 1997 was only 26 compared to 35 for the population as a whole (U.S. Bureau of the Census, 1998), reflecting this group's youth and high rate of growth. Yet the Latino population will age much more rapidly in the next few decades than will non-Latinos. The sheer number of Latinos 65 and over is expected to grow by 71% between 1997 and 2010 compared to only 17% for the older population as a whole. It is expected that an even higher rate of growth will characterize the decades beyond 2010 (U.S. Bureau of the Census, 1998).

As with many of today's older Latinos, a large proportion of the next decade's Latino elders will be poorly educated and have limited economic resources. Among the major race-ethnic groups, older Latinos have low average educational levels and the highest rates of poverty (Angel & Angel, 1997; Angel, Angel, Lee, & Markides, 1999). Unfortunately, poverty, limited education, and family disruption continue to plague minority populations, and many young Latinos will be unprepared to succeed in the 21st-century economy. As a result, many of tomorrow's older Latinos will become part of extended families with limited educational and economic resources. Although norms supporting intergenerational assistance are widely held in the Latino population (Burr & Mutchler, 1999), the support that these younger family members can provide may be minimal, and many may turn to their older relatives for assistance. Those young Latinos who acquire high levels of education and embark upon successful and lucrative careers–a growing share of the population–will be in a better financial position to offer support to elderly relatives. However, these advances may fragment traditional extended family norms as upward social mobility, and the geographic mobility that frequently accompanies it, increase the distance between generations.

Despite their poor socioeconomic profile, Latinos have lower mortality rates than Anglos in almost every age bracket (Markides & Coreil, 1986). Yet growing evidence suggests that despite mortality advantages, older Latinos, especially women, are more often frail and disabled due partly to a somewhat high prevalence of obesity and diabetes. Their health profile is further compromised by lower-than-average income levels and medical insurance coverage, resulting in limited access to health care systems. Yet, despite their disability and frailty, older Latinos seldom consider nursing homes. Perhaps this is why many Latinos, such as Puerto Ricans, shun institutionalization, ultimately entering nursing facilities with far more serious impairments than Anglos (Espino, Neufeld, Mulvihill, & Libow, 1988).

Although the majority of Latinos speaks English, language barriers are often substantial. More than a third of the Latinos aged 60 years and over speak English poorly or not at all (Mutchler & Brallier, 1999). More than one fourth live in linguistically isolated households, that is, households in which no one speaks English well. In health-care settings, language barriers between medical professionals and patients or family members may compromise accurate diagnosis, treatment, and patient compliance (Espino, Moreno, & Talamentes, 1993). The inability to speak and understand English well may also create a barrier to knowledge and use of other services and programs.

Researchers today not only recognize the importance of distinguishing between Latinos and non-Latinos in analyses, but also understand the need to differentiate among the major nationality groups, with each group retaining certain idiosyncrasies that are unique to its own culture and history in the United States. More than half of the older Latinos in the United States are Mexican American, and well over half of this group were born in the United

States (Angel & Angel, 1999). Only a small share–less than one fourth–is noncitizen. About one out of six older Latinos is Cuban-American, but very few of this group were born in the United States. More than half immigrated here during the 1950s, and fully half are not United States citizens. Puerto Ricans, constituting about 11% of the older Latino population, are a special case inasmuch as they are citizens of the United States; most have lived on the mainland for many years, albeit not necessarily on a continuous basis. The rest of the older Latino population is composed of a diverse mix of people from Latin American and South American origins, many of whom are U.S.-born and most of whom are United States citizens (U.S. Bureau of the Census, 1993). As a result of this diversity, many organizations will find that the older Latinos within their communities differ substantially from those in another community or the population reflected by national figures.

Based on this brief review, we argue that several characteristics of the older Latino population are particularly critical for public-policy analysts. First, issues relating to immigration and citizenship are important for significant segments of the Latino population. Policy focusing on the aging population must, by necessity, intersect with immigration policy and programs that treat citizens and noncitizens differently. Second, significant portions of the population will experience difficulty dealing with an English-only environment. Especially in those geographic areas where Latino communities are sizable, language accommodations are essential for the successful provision of services and information distribution. Third, due to shifting cultural traditions and demographic characteristics throughout the Latino population, traditional patterns of informal support by extended families may be difficult to sustain in coming years. Patterns of–and needs for–long-term care will be particularly affected by these changes. Finally, the intra-group diversity of the Latino population is considerable and must be factored into planning and policy development.

PROGRAMS SUPPORTING HEALTH
AND ECONOMIC WELL-BEING

Due to the economic and health profiles of the older Latino population, entitlement programs such as Social Security as well as means-tested programs like Medicaid are critical to the well-being of older Latinos. However, some aspects of the design of these programs have limited their benefits for this population.

Entitlement Policy

Social Security and Medicare are arguably the most important public resources provided to the older population, especially for those segments of it, such as Latinos, with few private resources (Angel & Angel, 1997). Yet rates of Social Security coverage by older Latinos in the United States are substantially lower than that of the general population (Chen, 1999; Social Security Administration, 1998). This is due partially to more frequent work in noncovered employment, intermittent work patterns, the holding of multiple Social Security numbers, and employers who fail to report contributions. Despite Social Security benefits, many elderly Latinos remain in poverty, or precariously close to it, and their retirement years are plagued by economic uncertainty. Moreover, a 1997 survey by the Pew Charitable Trusts shows that approximately one third of Latinos who are not currently poor fear poverty in old age compared with one fifth of non-Latinos, including Blacks and Anglos (Princeton Survey Research, 1998).

Although most older Latinos participate in Medicare, Latinos are more likely than others to report no health insurance coverage of any kind. In addition, older Latinos are more likely than non-Latino whites to rely solely on Medicare or Medicaid. Many report no Medigap or supplemental insurance coverage, largely due to its high cost. Any increases in out-of-pocket costs associated with Medicare will pose a particular hardship for those older Latinos with limited economic resources. As well, the large number of Latinos who rely exclusively on public insurance may have more difficulty finding a doctor, or may receive a lower level of health care services than others (Angel & Angel, 1997).

Immigration Policy, Welfare Policy, and Recent Reforms

For the past several decades, U.S. immigration policy has given preference to workers with needed skills and to family members of current citizens and legal residents. These policy outlines–along with refugee policy and the Immigration Reform and Control Act of 1986, which offered legal status to selected undocumented residents of the United States–have had important implications for the composition of the Latino population. Most of today's older foreign-born Latinos arrived in the United States as young people, participating in the work force for much of their adult lives. However, a significant number were admitted to permanent residence in the United States as elderly immigrants, most commonly as a parent of a citizen (U.S. Department of Justice, 1997). In general, immigrants face numerous social and cultural challenges in their transition to a new way of life, and often experience socioeconomic disadvantage as well. Indeed, the immigrant segment of the Latino older population has lower income and higher rates of poverty than the native-born segments (U.S. Bureau of the Census, 1993), and this is particularly true of those who migrate relatively late in life (Angel et al., 1999).

Recent changes in key means-tested programs have compromised the well-being of elderly immigrants. Welfare reforms over the last decade initially removed noncitizens from eligibility for most means-tested benefits, including Temporary Aid for Needy Families (TANF), food stamps, Supplemental Security Income (SSI), and Medicaid. However, food stamp and SSI eligibility have recently been restored to the elderly, and nearly every state has chosen to retain TANF and Medicaid eligibility for individuals who were already in the United States when the federal welfare reforms were enacted. Those entering the United States after welfare reform was passed (August 22, 1996) are still ineligible for these federal programs for five years. Recent immigrants are ineligible for many state-level programs as well, with some states imposing sponsor requirements in an effort to shift economic responsibility for poor recent immigrants to family members who sponsored their entry to the United States (Zimmerman & Tumlin, 1999).

These policy shifts are not directly applicable to the majority of older Latinos who are native born (48%) or naturalized (23%) citizens of the United States, although they may affect them indirectly through noncitizen family members. However, many older Latinos and their families have become caught up in a confusing bureaucratic web of shifting eligibility rules and barriers that often deter them from obtaining benefits for which they may be eligible. For example, some have failed to apply for benefits in the mistaken belief that they are ineligible for programs because of their sponsorship of family members' immigration in the past (Angel et al., 1999).

In addition, low-income families with minor children, citizens and noncitizens alike, have experienced the consequences of restricted eligibility for TANF. Because of these new restrictions, the ability of younger family members to provide support to aging parents may have been reduced. Indeed, these changes likely have resulted in increased needs for assistance from older Latinos by younger family members, both in terms of economic assistance and in-kind help (e.g., child care). And, although only a small number of elders serve as full-time caregivers or substitute parents for their grandchildren, it remains unclear how policies regarding eligibility and time limits apply to them (Wallace, Enriquez-Haass, & Markides, 1998). Above and beyond the financial strain experienced by those affected by these policy changes, the confusion and uncertainty resulting from this changing environment has had negative consequences for their mental and emotional well-being.

GOALS AND RECOMMENDATIONS

We close with several observations, goals, and recommendations regarding the needs of the older Latino population vis-à-vis the development of public policy. Although the social and demographic profile of the older Latino population is somewhat unique, a number of our recommendations have beneficial implications for members of other groups as well, especially other minority groups with large immigrant components. Some of our observations pertain most directly to the segments of the Latino population most at risk of health or economic disadvantage–the significant number of Latinos who live in poverty and are poorly educated, who do not speak or understand English well, who are not citizens of the United States, or who experience cultural or structural barriers to obtaining public benefits. Indeed, the need to take into account the diversity of the older Latino population is a crucial recommendation for policy and planning in the future.

A number of other recommendations and observations are noteworthy. First, the contributions of the Social Security system to the economic security of older Latinos must be protected or, ideally, expanded. Efforts to extend coverage to a larger share of this group would enhance the economic standing of large segments of this population, 27% of whom currently receive no Social Security benefits (Chen, 1999). As well, because Latino recipients are disproportionately dependent on Social Security as the major source of retirement income, it is particularly important that the "social adequacy" guarantees of this program be maintained. Plans to replace these guarantees entirely with individual investment accounts would hurt many low-income Latinos. Because there are no lifetime, inflation-adjusted benefits, the financial payouts of such a system would depend on the number of working years and earnings levels. Financially deprived Latinos have less to invest, due to lower-than-average lifetime wages and few private resources, and they would therefore receive lower benefits upon retirement. Less experience with investment markets would make this strategy especially risky for the uneducated segments of the population, including many Latinos. Innovations that combine the traditional "defined-benefit" provisions of Social Security with supplementary "defined-contribution" components, such as that proposed by Yung-Ping Chen (1999), should be examined with regard to their implications for low-income Latino elders.

We should start to redesign Medicare and other programs for the elderly in order to help families care for their aging parents when they wish to do so. Latinos' higher fertility levels result in larger families, and many adult offspring may be willing and prepared to care for their aging parents. In his 1999 State of the Union Address, President Clinton proposed an historic initiative to help families care for those relatives who need supportive services so that they can remain at home despite limited self-care capacities–the National Family Caregiver Support Program (NFCGP). The NFCGP is a $1,000 tax credit that would support the long-term care needs of approximately 1.2 million older Americans, 500,000 nonelderly adults, and 250,000 children. The program would also help those family members who care for and house their ill and disabled relatives. The plan is particularly valuable for the Latino population since it would complement, rather than substitute, formal supports for family caregiving.

We note that current Medicaid legislation potentially penalizes poor elderly Mexican Americans and others with large and involved families, such as those who have nearby adult offspring who would like to participate in the care of their frail parents. As part of the funding formula for the Primary Home Care/Family Care (PHC/FC) Program, states may restrict Medicaid or 1929(b) eligibility of nontechnical, medically related personal care services to functionally limited individuals who do not have access to other community-based services of support (Coughlin, Ku, & Holahan, 1994). Although physicians must prescribe PHC services, states also have the option to offer personal care services not prescribed by a physician to individuals at risk of institutionalization. Both PHC and FC services do not require the supervision of a registered nurse. PHC services include assistance with: (1) activities related to the care of the client's physical health, such as dressing and exercising, (2) household tasks that support the client's health and safety, and (3) trips to the doctor (excluding direct transportation of the client by the attendant). Although this exclusion was intended to limit participation to those with no other alternatives, it clearly discriminates against those who are most dependent upon their families. Rather than aiding family in caring for their elderly parents, this program may discourage this involvement. We propose, therefore, that the role of the family in providing care to elderly Latino parents be investigated more fully, with the objective of determining the best means of combining formal and informal care in the most cost-effective way. In our opinion, the effective use of the family as an adjunct in the care of the elderly could be enhanced by the selective use of targeted formal assistance, such as adult day care financed through mechanisms like Medicaid home and community-based service waivers.

We anticipate that more community and formal services will be required in coming decades, both because the older Latino population will be expanding, and because the intergenerational support system's ability to provide hands-on assistance will be weakened. Although intergenerational family ties are traditionally strong, many older Latinos live within extended families that are themselves undergoing rapid social and cultural change. Social and geographic mobility will modify the extent to which older Latinos can rely on informal networks to meet their needs for assistance. Greater opportunities for employment and schooling will erode the availability of future caregivers, especially the daughters who traditionally provide such care. As a result, more formal services will be required in the future (Torres-Gil & Villa, 1993).

For Latinos who have the financial means, long-term care insurance may be attractive. This product is poorly marketed to minority populations, and it is not affordable for low-income groups. Strategies for increasing knowledge and affordability should be developed. For example, some states are now considering support for long-term care insurance funds to which citizens can contribute–a strategy that would enhance affordability.

Aside from expecting more Latino clients, service providers will need to plan for needed accommodations in service delivery. An influx of Latinos into health and social service systems will require greater attention to culturally sensitive practices and efforts to overcome language barriers–changes that may mean providing training as well as a commitment to meeting the needs of a diverse population. Service providers who are aware of and sensitive to cultural heritage and possess specific knowledge about the subgroups with which they are working are required. Some organizations are moving in this direction. For example, a major HMO in the Boston area provides bilingual medical services at several health centers in order to improve the care given to the local major ethnic groups, and offers training in cultural competency to targeted providers and staff. However, most organizations have a long way to go. For example, although assisted-living facilities in Texas are affordable for wealthy Latinos, many do not provide culturally appropriate services and supports that might increase their attractiveness (e.g., offering Mexican foods, activities, bilingual nurse aides, etc.).

The well-being of today's as well as of tomorrow's older Latino population depends in part on the opportunities provided to its youth. Many of the problems facing this population stem from low average levels of education and income. Making certain that young Latinos are well educated and ready for the work force in the 21st century will benefit the Latino population as a whole (Chapa, 1999). Toward this end, the United States should invest in common and higher education for all youth, regardless of national origin or citizenship.

Finally, it is important for policymakers to understand that the patterns of service use over the past decade or two may not accurately predict demand in coming decades for the Latino population. This is a population in flux, a group that will continue to be modified not only by cohort succession but also by immigration and rapid social and cultural change. Organizations will need to be quick to respond if they are to effectively meet the needs of this changing population (Sotomayor, 1993).

Improving the well-being of older Latinos in the coming decade will require accommodation at all levels of government, as well as among private organizations serving elders. Meeting the economic and health-care needs of this population, for example, will require some retooling of the Social Security, Medicaid, Medicare, and public welfare systems. Some desirable changes include securing broad participation of the Latino population in these programs, facilitating the provision of culturally sensitive and linguistically accessible health care services, and removing the barriers faced by families who wish to care for their elders. Services for elders provided by all levels of government as well as by private organizations will be more useful if offered with sensitivity to the cultural and linguistic characteristics of the population. The contributions of private organizations may be particularly useful in aiding those segments of elders most under-served by governmental agencies: the sizable number of noncitizens as well as those citizens who are ineligible for many government programs. Finally, all organizations should take into account the fact that, because different segments of the Latino population are so unique, programs that target "the Latino population" will need to be customized at the state and local levels.

CONCLUSION

Issues surrounding the access of older Latinos to the major entitlement and means-tested programs are unlikely to be easily or readily resolved. Some are shaped by ideological interpretations of who deserves immigration to the United States, of citizenship, or of public assistance. Others are shaped by the stratification system in place in the United States, one in which resources are differentially allocated, disadvantage is passed on from one generation to the next, and the well-being experienced in later life reflects the opportunities experienced in youth. However, it is clear that the aging Latino population will be even more diverse in years to come, and that the new generation of Latinos will demand services and housing supports–such as retirement communities–that were once found unacceptable. Although Latinos vote less often than Anglos, the drawing of new congressional district boundaries that constitute a majority of Latinos could increase political power in their communities, and therefore trumpet a new political voice (Wallace et al., 1997).

One thing is certain: Acknowledging the policy options that hurt or help the health and economic well-being of elderly Latinos will inform the choices of our elected officials. Addressing the unmet needs of the elderly is too important to Americans of all ethnic identities and political persuasions not to deserve our concerted attention.

AUTHOR NOTES

Jan E. Mutchler is Associate Professor in Gerontology at the University of Massachusetts and a Fellow in its Gerontology Institute. She is currently conducting research on English proficiency and health behaviors among older Latinos, late-life labor-force transitions, and the influence of housing markets on intergenerational coresidence.

Jacqueline L. Angel is Assistant Professor at the Lyndon B. Johnson School of Public Affairs at the University of Texas at Austin. She holds a PhD in sociology from Rutgers University and is interested in social policy issues associated with minority aging, health, and long-term care, with special emphasis on Hispanic populations.

REFERENCES

Angel, J. L., & Angel, R. J. (1999). Aging trends: Mexican-Americans in the southwestern USA. *Journal of Cross-Cultural Gerontology, 13*, 281-290.

Angel, J. L., Angel, R. J., McClellan, J. L., & Markides, K. S. (1996). Nativity, declining health, and preferences in living arrangements among elderly Mexican Americans. *The Gerontologist, 36*, 464-473.

Angel, R. J., & Angel, J. L. (1997). *Who will care for us? Aging and long-term care in multicultural America*. New York: New York University Press.

Angel, R. J., Angel, J. L., Lee, G.Y., & Markides, K. S. (1999). Age at migration and family dependency among older Mexican immigrants: Recent evidence from the Mexican American EPESE. *The Gerontologist, 39*, 59-65.

Burr, J. A., & Mutchler, J. E. (1999). Race and ethnic variation in norms of filial responsibility among older persons. *Journal of Marriage and the Family, 61*, 674-687.

Chapa, J. (1999). Including Latinos in broadly shared prosperity. In R. Marshall (Ed.), *Back to Shared Prosperity* (pp. 103-109). Amonk, NY: M.E. Sharpe.

Chen, Y-P. (1999). Racial disparity in retirement income security: Directions for policy reform. In T. Miles (Ed.), *Full-color aging: Facts, goals, and recommendations for America's diverse elders* (pp. 21-31). Washington, DC: Gerontological Society of America.

Coughlin, T., Ku, L., & Holahan, J. (1994). *Medicaid since 1980: Costs, coverage, and the shifting alliance between the federal government and the states*. Urban Institute: Washington, DC.

Espino, D.V, Moreno, C. A., & Talamentes, M. (1993). Hispanic elders in Texas: Implications for health care. *Texas Medicine, 89*, 58-61.

Espino, D.V., Neufeld, R. R., Mulvihill, M., & Libow, L. S. (1988). Hispanic and non-Hispanic elderly on admission to the nursing home: A pilot study. *The Gerontologist, 28*, 821-824.

Markides, K., & Coreil, J. (1986). The health of Hispanics in the southwestern United States: An epidemiological paradox. *Public Health Reports, 101*, 253-265.

Mutchler, J. E., & Brallier, S. (1999). English language proficiency among older Hispanics in the United States. *The Gerontologist, 39*, 310-319.

Princeton Survey Research Associates. (1998). *Images of Aging: A Report of Research Findings from a National Survey*. Conducted for Americans Discuss Social Security (ADSS), Washington, DC.

Siegel, J. S. (1999). Demographic introduction to racial/Hispanic elderly populations. In T. Miles (Ed.), *Full-color aging: Facts, goals, and recommendations for America's diverse elders* (pp. 1-19). Washington, DC: Gerontological Society of America.

Social Security Administration. (1998). Why is Social Security important for minority groups. INTERNET: *http://www.ssa.gov/policy/pubs/bgpMinor.htm*, August 18, 1999.

Sotomayor, M. (1993). The Latino elderly: A policy agenda. In M. Sotomayor and A. Garcia (Eds.), *Elderly Latinos: Issues and solutions for the 21st century* (pp. 1-16). Washington, DC: National Hispanic Council on Aging.

Torres-Gil, F., & Villa, V. (1993). Health and long-term care: Family policy for Hispanic aging. In M. Sotomayor and A. Garcia (Eds.), *Elderly Latinos: Issues and solutions for the 21st century* (pp. 45-58). Washington, DC: National Hispanic Council on Aging.

U.S. Bureau of the Census. (1993). Census of population and housing, 1990: Public use microdata sample (computer file). Washington, DC: U.S. Department of Commerce, Bureau of the Census (producer). Ann Arbor, MI: Inter-University Consortium for Political and Social Research (distributor).

U.S. Bureau of the Census. (1998). *Statistical abstracts of the United States: 1998.* Washington, DC: USGPO.

U.S. Department of Justice, Immigration and Naturalization Service. (1999). *Legal Immigration, Fiscal Year 1997.* January. Washington, DC: U.S. Department of Justice.

Wallace, S.P., Enriquez-Haass, V., & Markides, K. (1998). The consequences of color-blind health policy for older racial and ethnic minorities. *Stanford Law and Policy Review, 9, 329-346.*

Zimmerman, W., & Tumlin, K. C. (1999). Patchwork policies: State assistance for immigrants under welfare reform. Occasional paper. Washington, DC: The Urban Institute. *http://newfederalism.urban.org/html/occa24.html.*

Time Not Yet Money:
The Politics and Promise
of the Family Medical Leave Act

Robert B. Hudson, PhD
Judith G. Gonyea, PhD

Boston University School of Social Work

KEYWORDS. Work/family issues, leave policy, Family Medical Leave Act, policy implementation, unemployment insurance

Robert B. Hudson is Professor and Chair, Department of Social Welfare Policy, Boston University School of Social Work. He currently serves as editor of *The Public Policy and Aging Report*, the quarterly publication of the National Academy on an Aging Society. Judith G. Gonyea is Associate Professor and Chair, Department of Social Welfare Research, Boston University School of Social Work. Her current research focuses on employment and retirement policy.

Robert B. Hudson can be contacted care of the Department of Social Welfare Policy, Boston University School of Social Work, 264 Bay State Road, Boston, MA 02215 (E-mail: rhudson@bu.edu).

[Haworth co-indexing entry note]: "Time Not Yet Money: The Politics and Promise of the Family Medical Leave Act." Hudson, Robert B., and Judith G. Gonyea. Co-published simultaneously in *Journal of Aging & Social Policy* (The Haworth Press, Inc.) Vol. 11, No. 2/3, 2000, pp. 189-200; and: *Advancing Aging Policy as the 21st Century Begins* (ed: Francis G. Caro, Robert Morris, and Jill R. Norton) The Haworth Press, Inc., 2000, pp. 189-200. Single or multiple copies of this article are available for a fee from The Haworth Document Delivery Service [1-800-342-9678, 9:00 a.m. - 5:00 p.m. (EST). E-mail address: getinfo@ haworthpressinc.com].

The Family Medical Leave Act of 1993 (FMLA) speaks in multiple ways as to how the American polity first acknowledges and then responds to social problems. The distal forces behind this legislation–demographic, gender, and workplace transformations in American life–might have been brought to-gether in a manner generating far more fundamental responses than were ultimately to be found in the FMLA. That they did not speaks to a host of more immediate political forces, involving issue definition, population and group involvement, and views of the appropriate role of government in American family life and in the American workplace.

The process of "policy minimalization" that is to be found in the FMLA case can be understood in different ways. In the classic "symbolic politics" formulation of Murray Edelman (1964), FMLA represents a widely heralded response but one that, in fact, calls for and marshals so little that it serves more of a co-optative than a remedial purpose. Or, invoking E.E. Schattsch-neider's (1960) construct of "the scope of conflict," the political resolution of FMLA was one where the potential interests of mass publics gave way to and were superseded by organized elite or "insider" interests, with the bias here being in favor of mutual accommodation rather than problem resolution. Finally, FMLA can be understood as invoking a "regulatory" rather than a "redistributive" approach (Lowi, 1964) to a broad-scale social issue: Rather than use public tax dollars to pay for workers' leaves, especially needed by low-income workers, FMLA followed the regulatory approach of mandating noncompensated leave policy on large employers only on behalf of noncon-tingent workers.

Both the construction and implementation of FMLA reflect these minimal-ist understandings of the American political process. Despite the fact that public discourse has been hot, key actors have been mobilized, and conflict has been sharp, major changes in the behaviors of either employers or work-ers are yet to be seen. In this sense, FLMA to this point has been "contained" legislation. But it does tap into fundamental beliefs about personal, private, and public responsibilities in ways that could be very interesting were they ever unleashed. Indeed, proposals in the fall of 1999 from both President Clinton and Democratic Presidential candidate Bill Bradley concretize the deeper appeal (and dread) FMLA conjures up among different parties.

FMLA AS AGE-RELATED LEGISLATION

FMLA is a curious piece of legislation insofar as the aged and the medical problems they disproportionately experience are concerned. The initial focus of family leave policy in the United States was on discrimination for reason of pregnancy, involving neither men nor the old, and the direct beneficiaries under current law are employees, not the frail elderly. Moreover, leave-taking for purposes of attending to the needs of an elderly parent–rather than for reason of the worker's or a child's illness–appears to have been slight to this point.

Nonetheless, there is an age-related logic to the FMLA approach to social policy that is very much worthy of note. FMLA benefits are directed toward the worker, but the purpose of those benefits is caregiving, that is, care *provision* provided by the employee to other family members. Among the FMLA care *receiving* family members, the aging parents of adult workers can be–at least in policy terms–understood differently than the other potential care recipients. While families have long taken care of their own–including aging parents, when necessary–such parents are the only "family population" for which major public care provision and financing programs are already in existence and on behalf of which there is much political pressure for further expansion.

Conceptually, at least, a greatly expanded FMLA would both reinforce family caregiving responsibilities and mandate an expanded role for the business sector in such activity. This may or may not be a good idea, but the logic of this approach connects long-term care coverage for the elderly and disabled to the workplace in a new manner. Juxtaposing this approach against more traditional social insurance mechanisms introduces a novel version of the "who should be responsible" question to the long-term care debate. In the language of John Myles (1986), should care provision fall to individuals in their private role as "workers," in their public role as "citizens," or be left, as has long been the case, to their informal role in "families"?

In light of FMLA's current modest status, posing these issues may appear to border on the ludicrous. But FMLA does serve as a useful vehicle for posing these broader questions. Moreover, the growing popularity of government mandates on private businesses and individuals means that these issues of respective public and private responsibilities are already on the table.

THE CONSTRUCTION OF FMLA

Leave legislation is about providing some modicum of security for workers who are allowed to temporarily leave work for an enumerated set of reasons. At its roots, leave legislation recognizes the intersection of work and family roles and the need to make some level of accommodation between the two. While tensions around work/family conflicts have and can be worked out at the bargaining table between employer and employee, involvement of government broadens the arena by constraining private behaviors or introducing public dollars.

At least in comparative perspective, discussion of "family policy" is of surprisingly recent origins in the United States. The concept of national family policy was not broadly promoted in the United States until the Carter

Administration suggested that the federal government should assure a more proactive role through the development of comprehensive programs to support families in the performance of their multiple functions in society. However, the 1980 White House Conference on Families, held during the waning months of Carter's term, was dominated by ideological disputes between conservatives and liberals centered on the definition of a family, passage of the Equal Rights Amendment, and the issue of abortion and reproductive choice. Policy options, such as those associated with work/family issues, could not surface in a forum where first principles about role and definition of core social institutions remained in play.

Ultimately, demographic pressures impinged on these ideological polemics and gradually moved the issue of work/family tensions into the political arena. Divisive issues still remained to be worked out, but the growing number of women in the workplace, the growing number of such women with young children, and, somewhat later, growing recognition of the number of workers with aging parents (Scharlach & Grosswald, 1997) provided a "numerical cover" that was not found in the broader heated debates about "the American family."

Family leave legislation first emerged in the case of the Pregnancy Discrimination Act in 1978, which banned discrimination against women for reasons of pregnancy, childbirth, or related medical conditions (Wisensale, 1997). Women's groups in particular favored broadening of the legislation for fear that limiting it to pregnancy and maternal care concerns might further stereotype the role and contributions of women in the workplace (Bernstein, 1997). During the 1980s, the debate broadened to parental leave for the additional purposes of child care to leave (in 1988) for purposes of assisting other immediate family members, particularly elderly parents as the aging of the population captured public attention.

The first iteration of a broadened FMLA reached the floor of both Houses in 1988, but died in the waning years of the Reagan Administration. A similar bill reappeared again in the early 1990s, but President Bush vetoed the FMLA of 1992, citing his opposition to the bill's strategy of imposing new statutory requirements on businesses. He offered instead the Family Leave Tax Credit Act, which provided for a 20% refundable tax credit to businesses with fewer than 500 employees that offered them up to 20 weeks of leave. Employers would have been eligible for a maximum tax credit of $1,200 per employee. Only with President Clinton's election did an FMLA bill become law in 1993, the first piece of domestic legislation that Clinton signed.

THE FAMILY MEDICAL LEAVE ACT

The key employee rights and responsibilities of FMLA are outlined in Table 1. Both a reading of the legislation and analyses of the politics behind it

TABLE 1. Key Provisions of FMLA

RIGHTS	RESPONSIBILITIES
Right to take 12 weeks of unpaid leave during a 12 month period for one or more of the following reasons: 1. Birth of a child and to care for the child 2. Placement of a child for adoption or foster care 3. Caring for a spouse, child, or parent with a serious health condition; or 4. Serious health condition rendering the employee unable to perform the functions of his/her position	Responsibility to provide 30 days notice that leave is needed if at all possible to do so Responsibility to provide notice of leave as soon as possible if 30 days notice is not practicable Responsibility to provide certificate from a health care provider of the need for leave if such certification is requested by the employer
Right to take leave intermittently or on a reduced schedule as needed	Responsibility to provide certification of fitness to return to work if requested by employer
Right to have his/her health premiums continued by employer on same basis as prior to commencement of leave	Responsibility to continue paying employee share of health benefit premiums if employee was required to do so before commencement of leave
Right to return to the same or equivalent position Right to same treatment regarding changes in employment conditions as employee would have been entitled to had leave not been taken Right to a reasonable period of time in which to become requalified for job if licensure, minimum hours of continued training, etc. is required by job and employee could not, as a result of being on leave, maintain that qualification	Responsibility to repay employer for employer's share of health care benefits if requested to by employer unless employee does not return to work because of: 1. Serious health condition; 2. Serious health condition of immediate family member; or 3. Some other reason beyond the control of the employee
Right to file a complaint with the Secretary of Labor if employer violates employee rights under the FMLA	

Source: Gowan and Zimmerman, 1996.

make clear the nature of the compromises that were necessary to ensure passage. Key here are the following: (1) no requirement for paid leave, (2) extending coverage only to employees who had worked a minimum of 1,250 hours during the prior 12 months, (3) limiting the duration of leave to 12 weeks (earlier versions provided for 18 weeks), (4) excluding small employers (earlier versions would have included companies with more than 20 employees), (5) restricting the need to medical conditions narrowly defined, and (6) restricting coverage to immediate family members rather than including extended ones as well. On the first item, it was with great reluctance but with equal certainty that the Women's Legal Defense Fund and the National Organization for Women acknowledged the legislative impossibility of enacting paid family leave (Elison, 1997). Yet, each of these restrictions–dealing with wages, length of leave, size of business, type of medical condition, definition of family caregiver–represented major concessions to bill proponents, to the point where some groups, such as the National Organization for Women, could not endorse the final bill. At best, such compromises ended up having to be judged "good politics" (Bernstein, 1997), if a bill addressing job *security*, incorporating gender neutrality, and covering a "life-cycle" range of family issues is considered reasonable progress.

To opponents, however, even the surviving provisions were problematic. In legal terms, a critique could be made that the FMLA is a "federally mandated exception to the common law concept of employment at will" (Aalberts & Seidman, 1996). At a more operational level, the most frequent concerns expressed by opponents were the increased costs and inefficiencies mandated family leave would bring to businesses (Scharlach, 1995), that it would depress wages for the very people it was designed to assist (Kosters, 1991), and that, philosophically, it would give government "the power to mandate . . . a benefit even if employers and employees do not want or need it" (Tavenner, 1991). In an earlier debate in 1987, the National Federation of Independent Businesses had raised the specter of "the Europeanization" of American labor policy, government imposing on American business new lists of employee benefits in the name of "the social good" (Sloan, 1987). Its members continued to lobby against FMLA in the 1993 debate, as they did in the case of the Clinton health care proposals, which surfaced during this period as well.

In the wake of the FMLA's passage, it remained to be seen if a federally mandated leave policy either would bring meaningful and secure relief to workers or create stifling anti-competitive pressures to businesses, or something in between.

IMPLEMENTING FMLA: PROVISIONS AND USAGE

The term used most frequently to describe FMLA's impact–on both employers and employees–is "modest." Of some import has been the substantial liberalization in employer leave *policy*, for example, extending the period of work absence, guaranteeing job reinstatement. And, among covered employers, formal eligibility for services is quite high–the Commission on

Leave (1996) study conducted by Westat and the University of Michigan found that 83% of those employees had worked the requisite 1,250 hours during the previous 12 months, although not all of these may have met the one-year job-tenure requirement. However, a notably smaller percentage of women are eligible for FMLA maternity leave; given restrictions and exclusions that are part of the law, the study estimates that only 19% of new mothers and only 31% of women employed one year before childbirth are eligible (Klerman & Leibowitz, 1994). Early estimates predicted relatively low *usage* of FMLA provisions. The GAO estimated that then-pending FMLA legislation would cost employers nationwide no more than $188 million, and of this total only $35 million would be lost to employers for reason of a seriously ill parent (*Congressional Digest*, 1991). Since passage of FMLA, usage has remained quite restrained. Thus, Scharlach (1995) reports on leave utilization studies showing leave-taking rates confined largely to only the 1% to 3% range of all employees, with somewhat higher rates among firms that continue to pay health benefits. In a University of Michigan Institute for Social Research Employee Survey conducted in 1995, two years after FMLA enactment, 17% of employees reported having at some point used leave for reasons included in the FMLA, but "just 7% of this group (or 1.2% of all employees) claimed that the leave was taken under the federal law" (Ruhm, 1997, p. 183). Finally, a recent case study undertaken by Grosswald and Scharlach (1997) of predominantly African-American women transit workers in northern California found that of the five qualifying reasons for leave-taking under FMLA–personal illness, new child, sick child, ill spouse or parent–the percentage of actual leave-taking was lowest in the case of ill spouse or parent.

Perhaps most notable is that the pattern of leave-taking that could have changed as a result of FMLA provisions has largely not. Among covered workers, 60% took leave for the employee's own health reason (other than maternity disability), 4% took leave for maternity disability, 13% for a newborn or adopted child, and 23% to care for an ill relative. But for workers in exempt establishments, the corresponding figures were 56%, 7%, 15%, and 22%, comparisons suggesting only minor impact of the law (Ruhm, 1997). And, as Ruhm goes on to report, while the ISR Employee Survey found that 17% of workers reported using leave for reasons that are covered by FMLA, only 7% of these workers claimed that the leave was taken under federal law.

The employee survey conducted by the Commission on Leave found younger workers (25 to 34) more likely to use leave than others, presumably because of the presence of infants in the family. Usage was also positively related to the presence of more children and higher incomes, the number of children representing potential need for leave time and the higher incomes representing the ability to take leave given that is usually without pay. The critical importance of paid leave is seen in data from the five states–California, Hawaii, New Jersey, New York, and Rhode Island–that provide Temporary Disability Insurance (TDI) to women on maternity leave. As a result of TDI, no low-income women in Rhode Island reported taking fewer than six weeks leave after childbirth (Bond, Galinsky, Lord, Staines, & Brown, 1991).

IMPLEMENTING FMLA: COSTS AND BENEFITS

Given the usage data, it is not surprising to find that benefits and costs ascribed to FMLA by both employers and employees have also been modest. Apart from occasional supervisory issues, Scharlach and Grosswald (1997) find employers reporting "no substantial" effect on costs of doing business. In the Commission on Leave study, well over 90% of establishments responding stated that FMLA had no noticeable effect on business performance or growth.

In fact, employers in the Commission on Leave study pointed to positive rather than negative business consequences from FMLA, including productivity (13% reporting positive effect, 5% reporting negative effect); turnover (5% vs. 0%); career advancement (8% vs. 1%); and ability of employees to care for their families (34% vs. 0%) (Ruhm, 1997). Salutary effects on employee morale may also be associated with family leave provisions, women employees in one study reporting being happier at their jobs and more likely to return to work after the birth of a baby, and employers in the University of California–Mercer study speaking of the beneficial effects of family leave policy on morale and on public relations (Scharlach & Grosswald, 1997). And Waldfogel (1999) points to the apparent positive if modest net employment effects of family leave policies pertaining to maternity issues.

While the latent demand for leave may be high among employees, relatively high levels of ignorance about the availability of leave and the fact that leave is almost always unpaid are major barriers to greater utilization. The Commission on Leave found that of those who were eligible for leave but did not take it, 64% cited financial constraints. Low usage of leave was found disproportionately among low-income, minority women. And while the possibility of leave may enhance employee morale, there remains the concern that taking leave may negatively impact one's job or career prospects (Scharlach & Grosswald, 1997).

FMLA: MUCH ADO ABOUT A LITTLE,
OR, A LITTLE ADO ABOUT A LOT?

Proposals to reform FMLA continue to tie modest programmatic outcomes to fundamental questions about the appropriate roles of family and government. From the left, the most fundamental proposal continues to harken back to paid leave. Thus, an analysis by the Institute for Women's Policy Research of state temporary disability-insurance programs concludes that "for less than the cost of the current Unemployment Insurance program, a new social insurance program could provide paid leave for family care" (Hartmann & Yoon, 1996, p.3). Democratic proposals build on the ideological edifice FMLA has precariously put in place, that is, the government has a legitimate social role in addressing employment-related tensions between employer and employee. These proposals would extend coverage to a domestic partner, parent-in-law, adult child, sibling, or grandparent if such individual has a serious health condition (bill introduced by Rep. Maloney of New York), extend coverage to employers with at least 25 employees (bill introduced by Sen. Dodd of Connecticut), and increase flexibility in use by allowing parents to take up to four hours in any 30-day period to attend or go with children or ill relatives for extracurricular activities or routine appointments (bill introduced by Rep. Clay of Missouri). By increasing the numbers of employers and employees subject to FMLA and by expanding conditions eligible for leave-taking, these amendments would significantly broaden coverage under FMLA. Presidential contender Bill Bradley has signed on to these Democratic proposals, calling for extending coverage to employees in firms with 25 or more employees and extending leave to nonemergency purposes, such as parent-teacher meetings.

On the right, there is no giving of ground in opposing such initiatives, as of this writing. Sen. Judd Gregg of New Hampshire and Rep. Harris Fawell of Virginia have pressed for clarify amendments to restore the definition of "serious medical condition" and "intermittent leave" to the original intent of FMLA (National Report on Work and Family, 1999). More fundamentally, right-wing commentators continue to question the basic premises of the law. Danielle Crittenden argues that liberals, in proposing expansions of the law, are undermining rather than supporting parenting "by paying mothers to care for their children for six months–but only six months–the Government would be setting a new norm: children are entitled to only as much of their mother's time as the state is willing to pay for." And, whereas Sen. Dodd is pressing legislation that would make parenthood a "protected class on the job," Ms. Crittenden argues that employer-based day care is frequently a hidden tax on other workers and sends a message that "you can bring your newborns right to the workplace . . . along with your briefcase" (Crittenden, 1999, p. 19).

In these arguments and proposals, we see yet again FMLA commentators lock onto both the fundamental and the modest. Where Crittenden would surely repeal the law, to say nothing of the thinking behind it, advocates for women, labor, and the old would surely break the existing mold by demanding *paid* leave for a wider array of family necessities. Remarkably, a proposal of President Clinton's would do that and more. His suggestion to use state unemployment insurance funds to support up to six months of paid leave for infant care represents a significant break with both the rationale and funding base of FMLA. Not only is supporting paid leave an important departure from FMLA history, but to locate the source of that support in unemployment insurance is conceptually enormous. Beyond being a basis for leave–even paid leave–infant care becomes a legitimate and supportable reason for not being employed. As such, the Clinton proposal is conceptually more daring than the state-based TDI programs currently in place, supporting infant care by associating such care with unemployment rather than disability status. Inferentially at least, the argument is not only that a woman is unable to work, but rather that she *or her husband* should not have to work even though their health status does not preclude it.

RECONSTRUCTING FMLA: NEW POSSIBILITIES

This article began by positing that the politics of FMLA might be seen alternatively in symbolic (Edelman, 1964), conflict (Schattschneider, 1960), or regulatory (Lowi, 1964) terms. Much of FMLA's history lends itself to interpretation in these terms. Symbolically, FMLA can be understood as having taken much of the wind out of the sails of IWPR and others to institute paid leave in America. Or, as Anya Bernstein (1997) nicely argues, the scope of involvement, and thus conflict, around FMLA's passage was limited largely to elite circles, thereby constraining both the range of options considered and the volume of mass pressure that might have been brought to bear on behalf of a more expansive program. And Lowi's regulatory politics, marked by zero-sum conflict around how to constrain (or not) the behavior of interested parties, certainly has been a central feature of FMLA passage and implementation.

Interestingly, the Bradley and Clinton proposals suggest at least the possibility that FMLA's politics and provisions could shake these intertwined understandings. Bradley may just be posturing (and Al Gore is on board with this type of expansion), but Democratic victories in the 2000 elections would almost surely lead to liberalization along these lines. And Clinton's major departure might end up being little more than a minor "last hurrah" of a departing president. Yet, paid leave, certainly coming from pockets as deep as those of the UI trust funds, would take FMLA beyond the symbolic. Should the UI proposal and expanding coverage to smaller employers gain credence, they would expand the scope of conflict around FMLA by involving a host of new actors, including both small business and organized labor. Finally, initiation of paid leave, especially were it through UI auspices, would extend

FMLA from Lowi's regulatory to his redistributive category, wherein notions of social class supersede those of interest groups.

This is all speculative, of course. But the Clinton proposal in particular does show how the latent ingredients always present in any family leave legislation where private employers are involved might be activated. More grandly yet, enactment of something along the Clinton lines would nudge U.S. social policy in the "citizenship" direction along the John Myles continuum. Unlike today's FMLA where one cannot lose a job for purposes of selected family-care activities, and unlike TDI-based liberalization where mothers are classified as disabled and supported while unable to work due to reasons of pregnancy and infant care, under the Clinton proposal parents would be identified as able-bodied citizens legitimately unemployed and therefore eligible for public support while not working.

The current political prospects of the Democratic party–perhaps reclaiming both the House and Senate while retaining the Presidency–and a new appreciation of work/family concerns that FMLA has long reflected now create the possibility that FMLA's future might find a central and contentious place in the 2000 election. Highly conflicted redistributive politics about real benefits would tilt the analytical firm of Edelman, Schattschneider, and Lowi in directions FMLA might once have promised but which it certainly has not delivered in its current form. Stay tuned.

REFERENCES

Aalberts, R.J., & Seidman, L.H. (1996). The Family and Medical Leave Act: Does it make unreasonable demands on employers? *Marquette Law Review, 80*, 135-60.

Bernstein, A. (1997). Inside or outside: The politics of family and medical leave. *Policy Studies Journal, 25*(1), 87-99.

Bond, J.T., Galinsky, E., Lord, M., Staines, G.L., & Brown, K.R. (1991). *Beyond the parental leave debate: The impact of laws in four states.* New York: Families and Work Institute.

Commission on Leave. (1996). *A workable balance: Report to Congress on family and medical leave policies.* Washington, DC: Commission on Leave.

Congressional Digest. (1991). *The Family and Medical Leave Act.* Washington, DC: Congressional Digest.

Crittenden, D. (1999, July 21). "A mother's place is . . . ," *New York Times*, A23.

Edelman, M. (1964). *The symbolic uses of politics.* Urbana, IL: University of Illinois Press.

Elison, S.K. (1997). Policy innovation in a cold climate: The Family and Medical Leave Act of 1993. *Journal of Family Issues, 18*(1), 30-54.

Gowan, M. A., & Zimmerman, R.A. (1996). The Family and Medical Leave Act of 1993: Employee rights and responsibilities, employer rights and responsibilities. *Employee Responsibility and Rights Journal, 9*(1), 57-71.

Hartmann, H., & Yoon, Y-H. (1996). *Using temporary disability insurance to provide paid family leave: A comparison with the Family and Medical Leave Act.* Washington, DC: Institute for Women's Policy Research.

Klerman, J.A., & Leibowitz, A. (1994). The work-employment decision among new mothers. *Journal of Human Resources, 29,* 277-303.

Kosters, M.H. (1991). Testimony on H.R. 2: The Family Medical Leave Act. Subcommittee on Labor-Management Relations, House Education and Labor Committee. Washington, DC. February 28.

Lowi, T.J. (1964). American business, public policy, case-studies, and political theory. *World Politics, 16,* 677-715.

Myles, J. (1988). Post-war capitalism and the extension of Social Security into the retirement wage. In M. Weir, A. Orloff, and T. Skocpol (Eds.), *The politics of social policy in the United States* (pp. 265-292). Princeton, NJ: Princeton University Press.

National Report on Work and Family. (1999). *Slants and trends.* Washington, DC: Business Publishers, Inc.

Ruhm, C.J. (1997). Policy watch: The Family and Medical Leave Act. *Journal of Economic Perspectives, 11*(3), 175-86.

Scharlach, A.E. (1995). *The Family and Medical Leave Act of 1993.* Boston: Boston University Center on Work and Family.

Scharlach, A.E., & Grosswald, B. (1997). The Family and Medical Leave Act of 1993. *Social Service Review, 71*(2), 335-59.

Schattschneider, E.E. (1960). *The semi-sovereign people.* New York: Holt, Reinhart, and Winston.

Sloan, J. (1987). The American folly of courting Europeanization: Benefits before business. *Vital Speeches of the Day* (February), 29-31, cited in E. Trzcinski (1994). Family and medical leave, contingent employment, and flexibility: A feminist critique of the U.S. approach to work and family policy. *Journal of Applied Social Sciences, 18*(1), 71-87.

Tavenner, M.T. (1991). Testimony on H.R. 2: The Family and Medical Leave Act. Subcommittee on Labor-Management Relations, House Education and Labor Committee, February 28.

Waldfogel, J. (1999). The impact of the Family and Medical Leave Act. *Journal of Policy Analysis and Management, 18*(2), 281-302.

Wisensale, S.K. (1997). The White House and Congress on child care and family leave policy. *Policy Studies Journal, 25*(1), 75-86.

TRANSPORTATION

How Will We Get There from Here? Placing Transportation on the Aging Policy Agenda

Roger W. Cobb, PhD

Brown University
Providence, Rhode Island

Joseph F. Coughlin, PhD

Massachusetts Institute of Technology
Cambridge, Massachusetts

KEYWORDS. Transportation, policy, technology, driving

Roger W. Cobb is Professor of Political Science at Brown University. Joseph F. Coughlin is Director of the New England University Transportation Center at the Massachusetts Institute of Technology.

Roger Cobb can be contacted care of the Department of Political Science, Brown University, Providence, RI 02912 (E-mail: roger-cobb@brown.edu). Joseph Coughlin can be contacted care of the Age Lab, Massachusetts Institute of Technology, 77 Massachusetts Avenue, Room 1-235, Cambridge, MA 02139 (E-mail: coughlin@mit.edu).

[Haworth co-indexing entry note]: "How Will We Get There from Here? Placing Transportation on the Aging Policy Agenda." Cobb, Roger W., and Joseph F. Coughlin. Co-published simultaneously in *Journal of Aging & Social Policy* (The Haworth Press, Inc.) Vol. 11, No. 2/3, 2000, pp. 201-210; and: *Advancing Aging Policy as the 21st Century Begins* (ed: Francis G. Caro, Robert Morris, and Jill R. Norton) The Haworth Press, Inc., 2000, pp. 201-210. Single or multiple copies of this article are available for a fee from The Haworth Document Delivery Service [1-800-342-9678, 9:00 a.m. - 5:00 p.m. (EST). E-mail address: getinfo@haworthpressinc.com].

Over the next 10 years the demographic profile of the United States will change to reflect a greater number and proportion of older adults. These adults will have transportation needs, preferences, and challenges different than any previous generations. Transportation policy, at all levels of government, should begin to respond now to anticipate the mobility demands of tomorrow's older adult population. Over the next 10 years transportation should be mobilized onto the aging policy agenda, affecting service providers and introducing technological innovation.

The ability to get from here to there is often overlooked. Transportation, the means to travel from point A to point B works so well for so many that it is ignored–that is–until it is no longer available. Transportation is the way that people connect with friends, family, health care, food, shopping, entertainment, volunteering, education, and the multitude of destinations and activities that make up an independent life. Clearly, older adults in the next century will require a variety of viable and seamless transportation options that enable them to remain connected to those people, places, and things that contribute to healthy aging. However, the current transportation system, and the institutions that manage and operate it, are unprepared to meet the mobility demands of the nearly one in five Americans who will be an older adult over the next three decades. The next 10 years present an opportunity to develop transportation policy for an aging society–one that will engage government, business, and individuals to set a new agenda, restructure institutions, and introduce technological innovation.

DRIVING INTO AN UNCERTAIN FUTURE

Most people, both young and old, define transportation as driving. The automobile for the past 50 years has been the mainstay of daily life in the United States. Receiving a driver's license at 16 or 17 years of age is a rite of passage to adulthood, freedom, and independence. Throughout life the license, and the ability to drive, become part of our personal identity defining what we can do, where, and when. Driving has certainly become more than just a means to travel between activities. It often defines who we are and our ability to remain independent as we age.

However, the natural aging process and the diseases that often occur in older age may conspire to reduce our ability to drive safely. The aging eye has difficulty recovering from the glare of headlights, seeing the road or other objects clearly at night, and distinguishing contrast and color of vehicles or signs. Reduced physical flexibility and strength may make getting in and out of a car more difficult and turning one's neck to see merging traffic problematic. Slower cognitive function may impair judgement about the speed and distance of vehicles as well as the reaction time necessary to respond to changing road conditions. For others, diseases such as arthritis and Alzheimer's or dementia may make driving difficult or, eventually, impossible.

As shown in Figure 1, which shows drivers between the ages of 25 and 74, the youngest and oldest drivers experience inordinately high fatality rates. While younger drivers (between 16-24) may experience fatal accidents due to poor judgement, older drivers, it has been argued, experience the second highest fatality rate due to their own personal frailty and inability to recover from a serious crash. The cause of older-driver accidents and fatalities continues to be both a research and a political question. What is uncontested is that the number of older drivers that have died on the nation's highways has increased. According to the U.S. Department of Transportation, the number of people age 70 and older killed between 1988 and 1998 increased from 3,716 to 4,934, or 33% (USDOT, 1998).

The number of older drivers today is far fewer than what can be anticipated in the coming decades. Forecasts that estimate future older-driver fatalities as principally a function of population growth suggest that the number of older-adult deaths may increase from about 7,000 today to 23,000 in 2030 (Burkhardt, Berger, Creedon, & McGavok, 1998). Figure 2 shows the projected growth in fatalities over the next three decades.

For some, driving is not an option throughout adulthood due to personal choice or impairment. However, the lifestyles of tomorrow's older adults are likely to be quite different than those of their parents. The characteristics and activity patterns of today's baby boomers–those born between 1946 and

FIGURE 1. Fatality Rate per 100,000 Miles Driven by Age Group, 1997

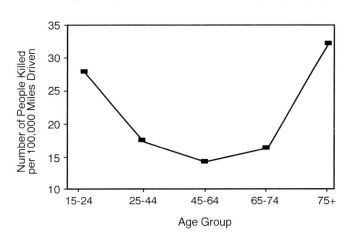

Source: USDOT, 1998

FIGURE 2. Projected Elderly Driver Fatality Involvement Rate, 1995-2030

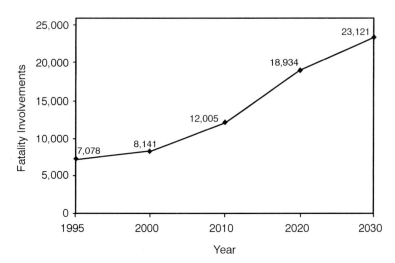

1964–suggest a more active older adult population with even greater transportation demands than previous generations.

GROWING MOBILITY GAP

Martin Wachs (1979) argued that older adults with higher incomes, better
education, and improved health would have higher travel demands than those
adults less fortunate. That is, education would provide a wide range of interests and income, and health would provide the capacity to pursue an active
lifestyle well into old age. Although not all older adults will be well off, a
larger proportion than ever before *will* be. Projections suggest that older baby
boomers will generally have more economic resources, education, and better
health than their parents.

The baby boomers represent the largest generation of double-income
households. Moreover, even if this generation does not save at the rate of
their parents over the next 20 years, they will inherit the single largest transfer
of wealth in history–nearly $14 trillion, increasing their disposable income
by nearly 29%. The number of older adults with four or more years of college
has doubled in the last two decades. Boomers will increase the number of older
adults with a college education by nearly 20%. Nearly 75% of today's older
adults report that they are in good to excellent health. Research also indicates
that disability rates among the elderly are on the decline (Singer & Manton,

1998). Improvements in nutrition, health care, and medicine would predict a generally healthier older population over the next 30 years.

In addition, changes in the behavior and expectations of women will influence future transportation needs. Unlike their mothers, boomer women have far more education, and many have pursued careers. The vast majority of boomer women drive more than their mothers and although they may not drive as far as their male counterparts, they make more trips as working mothers and caregivers. Boomer women will clearly have greater travel demands than their mothers.

Many surveys indicate that baby boomers fully anticipate pursuing a wide range of activities (Roper-Starch/AARP, 1999). One survey shows that older boomers are likely to pursue study, travel, volunteering, and part-time work well into their "retirement years." Boomers have enjoyed a level of unparalleled mobility and independence built mostly around the car. As they age they are likely to continue their pursuit of an active, engaged, and independent life that will rely on the mobility they enjoyed in their youth. Similar to previous generations of older adults, many boomers may find driving no longer attractive or a safe option–how will they, how will society, reconcile their demand for mobility with the capacity of the transportation system to provide it?

MEETING UNMET EXPECTATIONS

The current transportation system does not have the capacity to meet the needs of many older adults today–it certainly does not have the capacity to meet the scope or diversity of demands of tomorrow's older boomers. Although the automobile is becoming more technologically sophisticated, real focus on the older adult operator has yet to move beyond research by one or two manufacturers and development of several car models. For example, in addition to selected "intelligent system" applications such as enhanced night vision or collision avoidance, the physical design of the car should reflect the egress and ingress as well as safety needs of older adults. Industry should be encouraged to increase its investment in pushing the car to be a safe alternative for individuals for as long as possible.

Public transportation is the traditional policy response for nondrivers of all ages. However, public transportation in its current form is unlikely to provide a real option. More older adults than ever before live in the suburbs and rural America. Most boomers are likely to age in place as their parents are doing today–in the suburban and rural homes that are far beyond most public transportation systems. Where public transportation is available, many older adults have difficulty physically accessing the system while others perceive mass transit as unsafe.

Paratransit or demand-response systems that provide door-to-door service are growing in number. These services are more likely to meet the needs of older adults; however, they are currently expensive and difficult to provide, and are often operated as a "step-child" system to traditional bus and rail transit. Despite billions of dollars in federal and state funding, most paratransit services place a priority on providing transportation for medical and food shopping-related trips. Such systems frequently require at least 24-hour advance booking for health care trips and as much as seven days advance reservation for "other" trips. Planning a day's activities a week in advance is not a requirement in youth and it should not be in old age (Hudson, 1999). Healthy aging depends on being able to maintain social connections through entertainment, visiting a friend, window shopping, and a host of other activities that are well beyond trips to see the doctor and to buy food.

CRAFTING A NEW TRANSPORTATION AND AGING POLICY AGENDA

The inadequacies of the physical system reflect a larger policy and institutional problem. Most programs that support the transportation needs of older adults are based upon policy created more than 30 years ago. The definition of the "transportation problem" focused generally on providing necessary service to the poor and disabled. Although many older adults are poor and disabled, the majority are not. Moreover, the type of transportation needed by many adults today–and tomorrow–must be responsive to a different population, one that is more active and in many instances has more resources.

Policy innovation generally happens when events command the public's attention long enough to demand change. The glacial speed of demographics is unlikely to result in a single event that will trigger policy change in transportation for the aged. The other way innovation is introduced into policy is by a change of participants. In addition to the current interests that "own" the transportation and aging issue–state agencies on aging, community or area agencies on aging, transit operators–a number of other participants should be introduced to the debate.

These new stakeholders might include those with "an investment" in the mobility of older adults but who have yet to understand the scope of their interest. This includes health and long-term care insurers who pay when preventative care is missed or when social isolation results in depression and a spiraling down in well-being. Adult children provide much of the transportation that is not provided by public or private services. Businesses employ adult children who must take time from work to provide transportation, diminishing workplace productivity and contributing to caregiver stress. Financial planners who are used most often to plan for our financial futures might be encouraged to provide turn-key retirement services–to address the issues of transportation and housing. These may include a database of providers, financing strategies, and management of contracted services for individual users. For example, retirement fund managers and planners might become a service hub for older adults to purchase transportation services from private providers. In addition, many entrepreneurs are discovering the older-adult market as one that may have several lucrative niches. Some of these private investors might actually see markets in planning and providing alternative transportation services to those who might be able to pay for or co-subsidize transportation costs. These new players should be mobilized into the aging policy network to redefine how transportation is paid for and provided. Together, they might craft a number of policies that would help set the national agenda, spur real institutional change, and introduce technological innovation.

THE NEXT TEN YEARS

Table 1 outlines a number of activities that might be pursued by a new coalition of transportation and older-adult advocates over the next 10 years.

Agenda Setting

Both the government and industry have a role in placing the issue of transportation on the aging policy agenda. Despite its importance, it does not maintain a prominent position in policy deliberations in state legislatures or Congress or on the agendas of major aging interest groups. Government agencies and aging advocates must begin to educate the public and policymakers about the importance of transportation to older adults and the likelihood of a mobility gap in supporting the lifestyles of tomorrow's older boomers. Moreover, a national discussion should take place to determine the role and scope of public transportation in providing transportation for older adults. That discussion should include an assessment of current capacity and the adequacy of the resources available. This issue should then evolve into a larger discussion about how public policy might better serve the needs of all nondrivers–regardless of age.

Although important, transportation must compete with myriad other government priorities. Consequently, the public sector should consider adopting a social marketing strategy targeted at aging adults to bring attention to the need to plan for transportation–redefining mobility as a personal responsibility of individuals and families, not public transportation providers alone. Such a program could include a discussion of expanding the criteria of where to retire in the context of mobility options–retiring in the rural countryside

TABLE 1. National Transportation Policy Strategies for an Aging Society

ACTIONS / OBJECTIVES	PUBLIC POLICY STRATEGIES
AGENDA-SETTING	• Identify transportation as an issue for older adults. • Develop new data sets and tools to forecast and understand the mobility needs of a diverse older population. • Encourage a national discussion assessing the role and existing capacity of public transportation to meet the needs of an aging society. • Provide tax incentives for individuals to prepare for their transportation needs in later life and to industry to induce technological and service innovations.
INSTITUTIONAL CHANGE	• Shift focus from institutional coordination between public agencies (cost-effectiveness) to system coordination to provide seamless and responsive services (customer-focused). • Encourage multiple providers of transportation to respond to a diverse market while ensuring policy equity. • Craft relationships between other firms that may be able to provide services to individual markets, e.g., policyholders of a specific insurance firm.
TECHNOLOGICAL INNOVATIONS	• Invest in human factors research to better understand the unique physical and access needs of older passengers. • Adapt and integrate information and communications technologies to deploy a next-generation alternative transportation system that is responsive to all non-drivers. • Forge strategic alliances with the public sector to manage and operate networks of alternative transportation systems.

may be attractive, but what are the trade-offs if driving is no longer an option? Will a country home or a more urban choice facilitate continued access to social activities, health care, and shopping?

In addition, transportation must be placed on the agenda of individuals and families. As we plan for our financial and health futures, we must plan for mobility. Transportation accounts for almost 20% of household expenditures for those over 50 years old. Transportation planning should be a priority in retirement planning to ensure that we have the capacity to enjoy the benefits of good health and financial security.

Tax incentives for such planning may be the best way for it to achieve a prominent place on personal agendas. For example, the establishment of mobility accounts, to be used as those set up for pension savings, or "cafeteria" plans for eldercare, would encourage people to save before-tax income to provide funds for the needs of parents, spouses, transportation upon retirement, or when one no longer drives. A lifelong incentive to use these "mobility accounts" for transportation might include a tax penalty for use of these funds for purposes other than mobility, at least until one may become institutionalized. The use of the existing tax and savings infrastructure would ease implementation barriers and stimulate the development of a transportation market. It would spur private-sector services to respond to a growing social need and help ensure the continued mobility of adults throughout their lifespan.

Institutional Change

For nearly 30 years, efforts have been made at all levels of government to better coordinate public transportation and human services transportation. Medicaid remains the only federal program that guarantees older adults transportation access to medical services. However, the demand for these services has outpaced the availability of budget resources. Consequently, Medicaid, now focuses on "coordination" as a strategy to leverage other government resources and to control costs. The 1995 White House Conference on Aging recommended a number of actions regarding transportation–most of these involved coordination. The recently passed transportation authorization, the Transportation Equity Act for the 21st Century, also put renewed emphasis on coordination. However, most of these efforts have been focused on improved cost-effectiveness of operations, for example, eliminating redundancies in services or saving money. The Department of Health and Human Services spends more than $5 billion on transportation. Coordination remains important; however, the focus should be customer-focused. That is, how can we use existing resources to improve services to the older customer–not just control public spending?

The greatest change may be to actively encourage private providers to enter the older-adult transportation market to respond to the diversity of mobility demands and incomes. For example, firms that respond to other needs of older adults, such as entrepreneurs or insurers, could be encouraged to invest in providing transportation services. Clearly, public-sponsored programs are limited in their capacity to provide services to all segments of the older population. Public agencies might better serve as facilitators to leverage other providers–for-profit and not-for-profit–to enter the "mobility market." Government-sponsored transportation programs could then work with private providers to ensure equity for those who cannot afford certain private services.

Technological Innovation

Existing technologies offer great potential to improve the quality of transportation services that are available to older adults. In addition to research to better understand the challenges faced by older adults when using transportation, systems engineering and integration work should be conducted to fully leverage information and communications technologies. Wired and wireless communication could be used to integrate public *and* private providers into one regional mobility system for nondrivers of all ages. Similar to air traffic control systems used to manage multiple providers of air transportation, technology exists to manage seamless regional alternative transportation networks. Moreover, the revolution in easy-to-use, hand-held communication makes it possible for older passengers–and transportation providers–to remain connected and visible to each other wherever they may be.

The next 10 years offer a great opportunity to re-engineer the political coalition that influences transportation and aging policy for the next three decades. If we begin immediately, we will be able to introduce the institutional change and technological innovation necessary to ensure that tomorrow's older adults will be able to get from here to there.

AUTHOR NOTES

Roger W. Cobb is Professor of Political Science at Brown University. Joseph F. Coughlin is Director of the New England University Transportation Center at the Massachusetts Institute of Technology and leads MIT's new initiative in technology and aging, Age Lab (Technology for Healthy Aging Laboratory). Drs. Cobb and Coughlin are co-authors of a forthcoming book on the politics of older drivers to be published by Johns Hopkins University Press.

REFERENCES

Burkhardt, J.E., Berger, A.M, Creedon, M., & McGavok, A.T. (1998, July 4). *Mobility and independence: Changes and challenges for older drivers*. Bethesda, MD: Ecosometrics, Inc.

Hudson, R. (Ed.), (1999, Spring). *The Public Policy and Aging Report*. Washington, DC: National Academy on an Aging Society, *10*(1).

Roper-Starch Worldwide, Inc., and AARP (1999, Feb.). *Baby boomers envision their retirement: An AARP segmentation analysis*. Washington, DC: AARP.

Singer, B.H., & Manton, K.G. (1998, Dec.). *The effects of health changes on projections of health service needs for the elderly population of the United States*. National Academy of Sciences, *95*, 15618-15622.

U.S. Department of Transportation. (1998). *Traffic safety facts*. Washington, DC: Author.

Wachs, M. (1979). *Transportation for the elderly*. University of California Press.

Index

Aaron, H.J., 66
AARP. *See* American Association for
    Retired Persons (AARP)
AARP Public Policy Institute, 13
Achenbaum, A.W., 3-4
Achenbaum, W.A., 41
Administration of Aging, 130
Advancing aging policy, in 21st
    century, 1-6
Age
    as factor in FMLA, 190-191
    retirement, in Germany, increasing,
        61-70. *See also under*
        Germany
Aging
    advancing, policy for, in 21st
        century, 1-6
    of baby boom, politics of near-term
        action to deal with, 19-29
    in Germany, 62-63
    interest groups of, voluntary
        association as, 42-43
    of prison populations, dilemma of,
        168-171,169f
    of workforce, 83-88. *See also*
        Workforce, aging
Aging policy, transportation in,
    201-210
    agenda for, 207-209,208t
    creation of, 206-207
    institutional change for, 209
    policy strategies for, 207,208t
    technological innovation in,
        209-210
    unmet expectations related to,
        meeting of, 205-206
Aging society
    economic assumptions effects on,
        9-11

productive, moving toward, 7-17.
    See also Third Age
American Association for Retired
    Persons (AARP), 11, 45
American Medical Association, 142
American medicine, paradox of,
    107-114
Americans with Disabilities Act, 171
Angel, J.L., 6, 177
Austria, recent pension reforms in, 53

Baby boom. *See also* Baby boomers
    aging of
        addressing issues of, political
            factors against, 20-23
        as not immediate crisis, 20-21
        politics of near-term action to
            deal with, 19-29
        postponing action related to
            advance planning in, 23-24
        "crisis" as context for
            getting attention in,
            24-27
        distant startup in, 23-24
        enhancement of, 23-27
        gains vs. losses in, 21-23
        gradualism in, 23-24
Baby boomers. *See also* Baby boom
    behavior of, 11-12
    expected inheritances of, 12
    retirement age expected by, 11
"BABY K," 150
"Back to Basics," 78
Barth, M.C., 4,83
Bass, S.A., 3,7
Belgium, recent pension reforms in, 53
Bernstein, M.A., 198
"Beyond Social Security: The Local
    Aspects of Aging America,"
    13-14

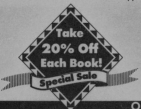
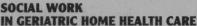